# Run for Good

## How to Create a Lifelong Running Habit

Christine Many Luff

Disclaimer:

The author of this book is not a physician and the ideas, procedures, and suggestions in this book are not intended as a substitute for the medical advice of a trained health professional. All matters regarding your health require medical supervision. Consult your physician before adopting the suggestions in this book. The author disclaims any liability arising directly or indirectly from the use of this book.

Copyright © 2018 by Christine Luff

No part of this publication may be reproduced or transmitted in any form or by any means, electronic or mechanical, including photocopying, recording, or any other information storage and retrieval system, without the written permission of the author.

Run for Good

run-for-good.com

*For Brad, Keira, and Brendan*
*My biggest cheerleaders in running and life*

# CONTENTS

## INTRODUCTION

## PART ONE: GETTING STARTED

**Chapter 1:** Why Start a Running Habit?.................3

**Chapter 2:** Tips for Getting Started......................9

**Chapter 3:** How to Dress Like a Runner...............15

**Chapter 4:** Tips for Proper Running Form.............21

**Chapter 5:** Treadmill Running Tips......................25

**Chapter 6:** 30-Day Beginner Running Program......27

## PART TWO: MAKE YOUR HABIT STICK

**Chapter 7:** Create a Habit Loop........................33

**Chapter 8:** State Your Plans............................45

**Chapter 9:** Plan Your Runs..............................49

**Chapter 10:** Practice Healthy Habits...................63

**Chapter 11:** Run With a Group.........................71

**Chapter 12:** Train for Races............................77

**PART THREE: OVERCOMING ROADBLOCKS AND SETBACKS**

**Chapter 13:** Be Prepared for Setbacks...................87

**Chapter 14:** Embrace Positivity............................91

**Chapter 15:** Bust Your Running Excuses.................99

**Chapter 16:** Prevent and Recover from Running...109 Injuries

**PART FOUR: GIVE BACK (AND RECEIVE MORE)**

**Chapter 17:** Ways Runners Can Do Good.............123

**Chapter 18:** Be Grateful......................................137

**Chapter 19:** Love Running – for Good..................139

**CONCLUSION:** Dos and Don'ts of Running...........141 Habit Formation

**RESOURCES:** Training Schedules for 5K, 10K.......144 Half Marathon, Marathon

**Suggested Reading/Bibliography**....................161

# INTRODUCTION

*"One run can change your day, many runs can change your life."*
-Unknown

Anyone can start running. Some people get excited about running, and they go out and buy new running shoes and expensive blister-proof running socks, or maybe even invest in a state-of-the-art treadmill. But those good intentions often fade as the running shoes get pushed to the back of the closet, the socks get shoved to the bottom of a drawer and the treadmill turns into a very expensive clothes hanger.

On the other hand, there are those people who start running and soon find themselves replacing their worn-out running shoes, socks and treadmill belt because of frequent use. They start to look forward to – and even begin to crave – their next run.

What makes the habit stick for some people and not others? Why do some people push through those first few weeks, maybe even months, of difficult runs to get to the point where they can run comfortably? How do you get to experience the life-changing effects of running?

Although I've been a runner for 30+ years, I'm not naïve to think that starting a running habit and, more importantly, *maintaining* it is easy. Doing any kind of exercise on a regular basis is really hard work. But through my work as a running coach for the past 15 years, my own personal experience as a runner, and the research I've done as a health and fitness writer, I've learned strategies and tricks to help break the cycle of starting and stopping healthy habits, then re-starting and stopping again, dropping your habit not too long after you've started.

## How to Use Run for Good

If you've ever wanted to get started with running and didn't know how to go about it, then this book is for you. If you've ever attempted to start running, did it for a few weeks, but just couldn't turn it into a regular habit, then this book is for you. If you're currently a runner, but feel like you could use some help in the motivation department and you're seeking expert running advice, then this is the book for you. Even once you've finished *Run for Good* and have an established running habit, you can re-visit it when you need some advice or a motivation boost.

While *Run for Good* details a lot of practical advice about getting started with running (what to wear, how to run, what to eat, schedules to follow and much more), it also explains the exact steps you need to take to establish a solid running habit and offers many habit-making strategies to make it stick. You'll get insights into why your efforts to start running, or any healthy habit for that matter, may have failed in the past and what you can do to change that pattern – for good. I'll also offer advice to help you make sure that roadblocks, such as lack of time and motivation, and obstacles such as injuries don't thwart your good intentions and undo your running habit.

Using the strategies and tips presented in this book, you'll develop (or re-discover!) a love and gratitude for running that will make you want to nurture and continue your long-term relationship with it. Think of *Run for Good* as an experienced, supportive and knowledgeable running friend, who wants to do everything possible to help you succeed.

## My Inspiration for Run for Good

I've gotten so much out of running that it's become my personal mission to introduce others to the sport and help them embrace it. For me, running has been both life-affirming and life-changing, and it has also helped to shape the person I am today. As a shy 12-year-old, running for my middle school cross country team boosted my confidence, physical fitness, mental toughness, and gave me a sense of community. Many years later, I still experience those same benefits from running, as well as many others.

Running has inspired me to reach goals I never thought possible and has helped me discover physical and mental strength that I didn't know I had. As a running coach of adults and young kids, some of my happiest and most satisfying running moments have been watching new runners triumphantly cross their first finish lines.

My positive experiences with running have inspired me to pay it forward and help others feel all the joy and positive benefits of running. I hope that this book encourages you to discover all the good things running has to offer, use running as a way to lift others up and embrace running as a lifelong habit. I hope that you'll be inspired to **Run for Good.**

**PART ONE**

# GETTING STARTED

*"You don't have to see the whole staircase.
Just take the first step."*
-Martin Luther King, Jr.

# Chapter 1
# Why Start a Running Habit?

*"I run because if I didn't, I'd be sluggish and glum and spend too much time on the couch. I run to breathe the fresh air. I run to explore. I run to escape the ordinary. I run... to savor the trip along the way. Life becomes a little more vibrant, a little more intense. I like that."*
-Dean Karnazes, ultra-marathoner and author

I love to ask beginner runners why they want to start running because the answers are always so varied. I hear things such as, "I want to improve my health." "I want to lose weight." "I want a challenge." When people give their reasons, I often ask, "And what else?" I like to encourage runners, especially new ones, to find many different motivations for running because usually one reason just isn't going to cut it. For example, if weight loss is the ultimate goal, what happens when the weight doesn't immediately start falling off like you had hoped? Will you still be motivated to run? You'll need other inspirations to keep you going.

I've been running for more than 30 years and, although many of my reasons (fitness, camaraderie, reaching goals) for running have stayed consistent over the years, I've added a bunch of new ones along the way. After I had my two kids, I wanted to be a healthy role model for them and make sure I was around for them for a long time. Oh, and running helps me stay sane when trying to manage all the challenges, crazy stress and drama that come with raising two young children. I tell my husband, Brad, and our kids all the time that my running habit makes me a much easier person to live with.

To make a lasting change or start a habit that endures, we need to have a sense of purpose. In their book *The Power of Full Engagement: Managing Energy, Not Time, Is the Key to High Performance and Personal Renewal* (which I highly recommend to anyone looking to make positive life changes), authors Jim Loehr and Tony Schwartz write: "In the face of our habitual behaviors and our instinct to preserve the status quo, we need inspiration to make changes in our lives."

Once you determine and define your reasons for wanting to start a running habit, you'll feel much more engaged in the process. Your purpose for running will help fuel you as you get started, especially during the first few critical weeks of habit formation. And when your running habit inevitably hits some rough patches and obstacles, your inspiration will help guide you through the storms.

Maybe you started this book thinking you only had one or two reasons why you want to start and maintain a running habit. But I bet you could easily embrace several more. Check out these benefits of running for even more reasons to love the sport.

**1. You'll improve your health.** One of the biggest and most commonly mentioned benefits of running is that it's good for your health. Regular running strengthens your heart and ensures the efficient flow of blood and oxygen throughout the body, which help decrease your heart attack risk. Exercise, combined with maintaining a healthy weight, is one of the best ways to naturally reduce high blood pressure and cholesterol. Running also boosts your immune system, so your body is more effective and efficient at fighting off germs. As a weight-bearing exercise, running increases bone density, which can prevent osteoporosis.

**2. You can lose weight.** Many people start running with the goal of shedding some pounds, or maintaining their current weight. As one of the most vigorous exercises out there, running is an extremely efficient way to burn calories and lose or maintain weight.

Many runners find that once they establish a running habit, the discipline, focus, and motivation they get from running leads to healthier eating habits and eventually weight loss. Running becomes a "keystone habit" (which we'll talk about more later in this book) that has a positive effect on other areas of a runner's life.

**3. You can train for a specific goal.** Training for a race gives you a specific goal to work toward, which can definitely help improve your motivation to exercise. Those who have had prior problems with "exercising just for the sake of exercising" often have more success with running, as they set running goals and train for races.

**4. You can experience something new and different.** Running is a great way to expand your horizons and switch up your normal routine. Through running, you can explore new locations and experience new physical sensations. You can always keep it interesting by trying new routes, participating in different races, running with friends, and doing new workouts.

**5. You'll sleep better.** Runners find that the more they run, the more their bodies crave sleep since it repairs itself while you're resting. Research confirms that exercise can help you sleep better.

Researchers at Stanford University School of Medicine asked sedentary adults suffering from insomnia to exercise for twenty to thirty minutes every other day in the afternoon. They found their time required to fall asleep was reduced by half, and sleep time increased by almost one hour.

**6. You can do it practically anywhere.** You don't need to travel somewhere to run – just head out your front door and go for a run. If you're traveling, it's easy to pack your running shoes and clothes in your suitcase. And running is a fun, interesting way to explore a new destination. Whether you prefer wooded trails, the beach or the mountains, it all serves as a peaceful backdrop for running.

**7. You'll feel more energetic.** When you're feeling sluggish, running is a great way to boost your energy. Indeed, a 2012 study in the *Journal of Adolescent Health* proved that just 30 minutes of running during the week for three weeks boosted mood and concentration during the day.

**8. You'll get stress relief.** The mental benefits of running are tremendous. Running gives you a break from the pressures and stresses of everyday life. Going for a run can help you clear your mind, problem-solve without getting too emotional and put things into perspective. What feels like an insurmountable problem somehow just doesn't seem like a huge deal after a run.

**9. You can get the whole family involved.** Running is a great way for families to spend time together. Family members often run and do races together. If some relatives don't want to run races, the non-running members can cheer or volunteer. I often run alongside my kids as they ride their bikes and scooters, or roller-blade. Even if they're not running, we're still having fun being active together.

**10. Running is cheap!** Unlike other sports that require expensive gear, running requires very little equipment. You don't even need a gym membership. All you need is a good pair of running shoes and you can head out your door to go for a run.

**11. You can make a difference.** Running is an excellent way to contribute to your community and beyond. Many races benefit non-profit organizations, and some charities offer race training in exchange for fundraising. Running for something that's bigger than you is a great way to stay motivated to keep training and can make running feel more meaningful and fulfilling.

**12. You'll feel good about yourself.** People who run on a regular basis report an increase in their confidence and self-esteem. You'll get an even bigger self-esteem boost when you accomplish a specific goal, such as running a 5K. The mental benefits of running will undoubtedly spill over into other areas of your life. Many runners I know are more productive at work or become more active socially once they establish a running habit.

**13. You can run by yourself – or with others.** Unlike other sports that can't be played alone, running can be a perfect solo activity. But if you love to socialize and get motivated by other runners, you can always run with a friend, join a running group, or participate in a race.

**14. You'll add more structure and discipline to your life.** As you develop a running habit, your runs will become focal points in your week. You'll plan other activities around them, and your days will have more structure. You'll also become more disciplined, especially if you decide to follow a training schedule. Your improved organizational skills and discipline will help you achieve other goals unrelated to running.

**15. You'll be part of the running community.** The sense of community and camaraderie among runners first attracted me to running and it continues to be one of the major reasons why I'm so passionate about the sport. Running allows people to come together to help others, whether it's encouraging one another to reach goals, raising money for causes or making a difference in their community.

Runners develop bonds that go deep and they support each other in running and many other areas of their lives. They have a common interest and shared experiences that allow them to connect on so many levels. When some runners struggle to stay motivated, it's often members of their running community who hold them accountable and pull them through the rough patches.

## What's Your Motivation?

So I've just mentioned lots of running benefits, but I've got plenty of other motivations to run. Here are some more:

- Running makes me feel free.
- I love finish lines.
- I want my kids to be active.
- I love exploring new places through running.
- Runner's high
- I really like dessert.
- Running makes me feel calm.
- I love being in nature.
- I think more creatively when I run.
- I love being part of a team.
- I'm more focused when I run.

- I like to burn calories efficiently.
- I like spending time with friends who also run.
- I like other runners. I even married one.

## Grab a notebook!

Throughout this book, I'll be suggesting simple activities to help you with your running habit formation. Some of them require jotting down some notes, so it'll be helpful to have a notebook (or computer/phone) to keep your notes and thoughts in one place. Many runners like to record their workouts in a training journal, so you can also use the notebook to keep track of your progress.

Here's your first (very simple!) assignment:

## TO DO: Write Down Your Reasons

Why do YOU want to run? I bet you could think of plenty of reasons that are personal to you and your situation.

Write down your reasons for running as a constant reminder of why you want to keep running. Keep revisiting your list to remember why you want to keep running and to add even more reasons.

Think about your reasons every time you start a run. When you face obstacles and setbacks related to your running habit, which we'll discuss later in this book, re-read all those reasons why you get started in the first place.

# Chapter 2
# Tips for Getting Started With Running

*"Anybody can be a runner...We were meant to move. We were meant to run. It's the easiest sport."*
-Bill Rodgers, four-time winner of the Boston Marathon

Running is so simple – just tie your shoes and start, right? Yep, it's sounds pretty easy but, in reality, getting started with running can feel quite intimidating to some people. What should I wear? Can I walk? What do I do with my arms? I feel awkward! Are people going to be staring at me?!

Even if you've run before, you may feel like you've forgotten everything you learned, lost all that fitness you worked so hard to build up and are starting over.

Some people give up on running because they feel overwhelmed by all the questions or it just seems, well, hard. So laying the groundwork and acquiring some essential knowledge about running are crucial to establishing a fulfilling, lifelong running habit. Think of it as getting started on the right foot. (Pun intended.) Here are some key tips to get you going.

**Get a medical check-up.** Planning to start a new running routine is the perfect excuse to visit your doctor. While you may not think it's necessary, if you're a man over age 45 or a woman over age 55, and especially if you have a family history of heart disease or you have an existing medical condition, you should definitely get your doctor's clearance. At your doctor's visit, share your running plan and goals with your doctor and have him/her assess your plan and any potential health issues. Ask how running might affect any existing conditions.

**Start small with mini habits.** New runners can be pretty ambitious and often start out running too much, too soon, too hard. Don't jump into a running habit thinking you're going to train for a marathon in a few months. This approach often leads to injury, running burnout or boredom, and can cause an enthusiastic new runner to throw in the towel.

It's extremely important for beginner runners to start out with realistic, manageable goals. Think baby steps. Starting out with reasonable, small goals – like running for 20 minutes consistently – will make it easier to stick to your running plan in the first few critical weeks as you start to establish your running habit.

No goal is too small as a starting point. You can start out by aiming to run or run/walk for five minutes or even just one minute a day. Whatever your fitness level, pick a starting point that works for you. Just keep it very simple. And easy. You want to make your mini running habit so easy that it's difficult to fail. By setting an achievable, easy starting point, you'll always hit your target, and sometimes surpass it, so you won't face those feelings of guilt or inadequacy that kick in when you fail to stick to an ambitious goal.

**Use the run/walk method.** For new runners, the best approach is to use a run/walk strategy, where you alternate between intervals of walking and running to build up your running endurance. The running schedule later in this section uses that method. Try intervals of running for one minute, then walking for one minute. If that's too easy, add more minutes to your run intervals. Continue to increase your run intervals as you build up your endurance.

If your goal is to eventually run continuously – don't worry – you'll slowly build the fitness and confidence to run long without walk breaks. And don't beat yourself up about walking for part of the distance. There are lots of benefits to a run/walk approach, and many experienced runners incorporate walk breaks into their training runs and races to improve their endurance and avoid injuries.

**Always start with a warm-up.** No matter what type of run you're doing, it's important to warm-up beforehand to get the blood flowing and make sure your muscles are warmed up for exercise. By slowly raising your heart rate, the warm-up also helps minimize stress on your heart when you start your run.

Your warm-up can be a 5-minute brisk walk or a slow jog, or warm-up exercises such as jumping jacks, knee lifts, arm and leg swings, marching in place or butt kicks.

**Take it easy.** Many running injuries are a result of overtraining: too much intensity, too many miles, too soon. Some new runners get excited and try running every day. That's perfectly fine if you're starting with a mini habit, such as running for five minutes each day. But if you're running a few miles each time, you need to incorporate days off into your schedule. Even the most experienced runners need at least one, even two, days off from running a week. Research has shown that taking at least one day off a week reduces the frequency of overuse injuries. Your body will have a chance to recover and repair itself, and you'll actually feel better during your runs.

If you're just getting started with running, you may want to run every other day, to give yourself enough recovery time. You can take a complete rest day or do a cross-training activity.

And don't increase your weekly mileage by more than 10% each week. You can still push yourself, but be patient and take a gradual approach. Use common sense and a smart training schedule to decide how much you should be running.

**Breathe from your belly.** Taking deep breaths from your belly while you're running will allow you to take in more oxygen and help you avoid side stitches. Deep belly breathing also helps reduce anxiety, so you'll feel more relaxed as you're running. Follow these tips:

• To do deep belly breathing, take a deep breath in and push your stomach out while pushing down and out with your diaphragm. If your upper chest is expanding, you're breathing too shallow. You should be breathing in through your mouth and nose, to get the most amount of oxygen.

• You should exhale through your mouth and try to focus on exhaling fully, which will remove more carbon dioxide and also help you inhale more deeply.

- Try to take three footstrikes for every inhale, and two footstrikes for every exhale. So, as you step, left foot, right foot, left foot, count, "1, 2, 3" to yourself.
- As a beginner, try to run at a pace at which you can breathe easily. Use the "talk test" to figure out if your pace is appropriate. You should be able to speak in full sentences, without gasping for air.
- Slow down or walk if you're running out of breath. If you relax and slow the pace, breathing problems often take care of themselves. Don't overthink it!

**Listen to your body.** Pay attention when something just doesn't feel right. If you're feeling sluggish, achy or lightheaded, it might be a sign of overtraining, a potential injury or a nutritional deficiency. Don't just ignore it. If something doesn't feel right, take a rest day. Talk to your healthcare professional if symptoms persist.

**Aim for 180 steps per minute.** Many new runners start out taking long, heavy strides, which can increase your injury risk. Running with quick, short steps uses less energy than long strides and decreases the stress on your muscles. The slower your stride turnover, the longer you spend in the air. As a result, you'll hit the ground with much greater force. So a quicker turnover means less impact on your joints.

You can determine your stride count (also known as cadence) by timing yourself for a minute, counting how many times one foot hits the ground, and then multiplying by two. Ideally, you want to aim for 180 steps per minute, which is an efficient stride count. However, that might be too ambitious for new runners. So try shooting for 170 steps per minute and work to gradually improve it.

To increase your stride turnover rate, focus on taking quick, light steps. Pick your feet up as soon they hit the ground, as if you're stepping on hot coals. Think to yourself, "Light on my feet, light on my feet." You should feel like you're gliding over the ground, not plodding. Be careful not to overstride. Your feet should be landing under your hips, not in front of you.

Doing running drills such as butt kicks, skipping, high knees, running backwards or side shuffles is another way you can work on improving your turnover, since you need to be light on your feet and turn over quickly as you're doing them.

As you improve your stride turnover, you'll also find yourself feeling more comfortable and less fatigued when running longer distances.

**Don't eat immediately before a run.** Many new runners wonder what and when they should eat before running. When you begin a run, you should feel neither starved nor stuffed. You don't want to eat immediately before running because it may lead to cramping or side stitches. But running on a totally empty stomach may cause you to run out of energy and leave you feeling fatigued and lethargic during your runs. Your best bet is to eat a snack or light meal about 1 1/2 to 2 hours before you start running.

Examples of some good pre-run meals or snacks are a banana and yogurt, a bagel with peanut butter, or cereal and milk. Avoid anything greasy or high in fat, as it may lead to gastrointestinal distress during your run.

# Chapter 3

# How to Dress Like a Runner

*"Life is better in running shoes."*

I started running as a kid in the 1980s before hi-tech, wicking running clothes and fancy running shoes were all the rage. I typically ran in cotton T-shirts and shorts, cotton socks, and a pair of beat-up Etonic sneakers.

Nowadays, runners have so many options for running clothes and shoes that shopping for gear can be pretty overwhelming. Runners who I coach often ask questions like, "What kind of running shoes do YOU wear?" "What are the best brands for running shorts?" "What sports bra should I wear?" The answer to all of those questions – much to the frustration of runners who just want simple answers – is, "It depends."

Like with many things in running, what's good for one runner may not necessarily work for others. I've been running in Mizuno Wave Riders for more than 10 years, but Brad swears by his Brooks Adrenaline. So, it's tough to give specific brand recommendations for clothes and shoes.

However, there are certain features that I suggest you look for when shopping to make sure you find clothes, shoes and gear that will help you feel comfortable and confident when you hit the roads.

It's important for your running shoes and clothes to feel and look right because you don't want "my shoes are too uncomfortable" or "my sports bra doesn't fit right" to be excuses or obstacles for your running habit.

Following are tips on how to choose the right running shoes, shirts, socks, sports bras and shorts.

## Running Shoes

If you're only going to invest in one piece of running gear, make it a good pair of running shoes. Finding the right running shoes for you is critical because wearing old ones or shoes that aren't right for your foot type and running style can lead to injuries, foot blisters, black toenails (ouch!), discomfort during runs and all kinds of other issues.

Some new runners give up on a running habit because they think they're just "not built to be a runner" when, in reality, they're just wearing the wrong running shoes.

Even if you have an old pair of running shoes that you think are comfortable, the cushioning may be worn out, so they most likely need to be replaced. You need fresh, well-cushioned shoes that are designed for running, fit well and are appropriate for your foot type and running style. If you have high arches, for example, you need a different type of shoe than someone who has flat feet.

Visit a running specialty store, where experts can evaluate your foot and running gait and make recommendations for the right shoes for you. The shoe expert will probably give you a few different options to choose from. He or she should have you test them out on a treadmill or running outside the store. Once you find a pair of running shoes that work for you, be sure to replace them every 300 to 400 miles because the cushioning will start to wear out.

## Running Shirts

It's best to run in shirts made from a wicking material, so the fabric pulls the moisture away from you and dries quickly. That means don't run in cotton shirts, which stay wet once they're wet. Look for flat seams to avoid painful chafing and discomfort. Reflective stripes or piping are another useful feature, especially if you tend to run in low-light conditions. Other desirable, although not totally necessary, features include UV-protective coating for increased sun protection and anti-odor technology.

## **Running Socks**

Shopping for socks can be confusing because there seem to be tons of options and a lot of them look pretty similar. So what are we looking for? As with running shirts, when buying running socks, the most important feature is the material. You'll want to stay away from 100% cotton socks, which don't wick away moisture. Running in socks that are wet from sweat or puddles can lead to blisters. And if it's cold out, your feet will feel cold and clammy.

The best running socks are ones that are made from synthetic materials such as polyester, acrylic and CoolMax because they'll wick away moisture. For cold weather running, wool blends such as SmartWool are also an excellent choice.

Other features to look for are seam-free toe section (for more blister protection) and an elastic arch lock (to keep the sock in place). Padded soles are also good to give you some heel cushioning. If you like low-cut socks, make sure that they have a tab that covers your Achilles, so your running shoe isn't digging into or irritating your skin. And if you plan to do some trail-running, look for ankle socks (rather than low-cut) to keep tiny pebbles out of your socks and shoes.

## **Running Shorts**

Look for running shorts with an elastic waistband and a thin liner for comfort and to hold everything in place. Another great feature is a small pocket, where you can store your keys, ID or nutrition. As with running shirts, some reflective piping or stripes for early morning or evening running is always a plus.

**Tips:** Once you find a pair of comfortable running shorts, capris or pants that you absolutely love, get another pair of them. You don't want to let "my favorite shorts are in the laundry" be an excuse to skip your run. Also, running clothes and shoes are sometimes discontinued, so it pays to stock up on your favorites before they're impossible to find. I still kick myself for not buying another pair of my absolute favorite capris before Brooks stopped selling them a few years ago.

## Sports Bras (for the ladies!)

A good, supportive sports bra can immensely improve female runners' comfort and confidence while running. Your sports bra should fit you properly and not be too stretched out. Most sports bras need to be replaced after about 72 washes, if you've had a significant weight change or the bra's elastic is shot. So if you've been holding onto your favorite sports bra for a while, buy the same brand/model and retire the old one.

Your best bet is to go to your local running specialty store for a sports bra, since they'll have bras that are designed specifically for runners and the salespeople can give you some expert advice. Many sports bras don't have the right support for runners, especially if you're large-chested. Follow these sport bra shopping tips to ensure the right fit:

• Make sure you try the sports bras on, in several different sizes. The right size for you may not actually be your usual size. You'll know that the bra is too big if the material wrinkles or bunches.

• The bra should be snug, but not too small or tight. It should fit snugly but not constrict your breathing or dig into your skin. It's a good fit if you can slide two fingers under the straps.

• Avoid sports bras that are made of 100% cotton because once you start sweating, they'll stay wet and that could lead to chafing and general discomfort. Look for moisture-wicking fabrics such as Coolmax and Drifit.

• Rough seams can also cause chafing. Look for seamless fabrics, seams with rolled edges, or covered seams.

• When you're trying on sports bras, jog in place or jump up and down to test their support. The bra should minimize breast movement as you're bouncing.

• If you have a large chest and need a lot of support, look for sports bras with wide shoulder straps and racer back straps. A few brands that specialize in sports bras for runners with large chests are Enell, Shock Absorber and Brooks (formerly Moving Comfort).

## TO DO: Get fitted for running shoes and (ladies) a good sports bra

These are two of the most important steps you can take to get your running habit started. By investing some money on one or two key pieces of running gear, you'll feel like you have some skin in the game and be more motivated to get started. Lacing up your running shoes will start you on the road to feeling more like a runner.

## How to Get Over Feeling Self-Conscious About Running

*"I really want to start running, but I feel too self-conscious to run, especially outside in my neighborhood. How do I get over this?"*

You're not alone – fear of being seen running on the roads or even on a treadmill at the gym keeps a lot of people from starting or continuing a running habit. You may be worried that you'll look slow, silly, too fat, too old to other runners or people driving by.

**Don't be concerned about what others think!** As a runner, you deserve respect from other runners. Besides, runners love seeing others out on the roads or trails. We know how much enjoyment we get out of the sport, so why wouldn't we want to see other people doing the same thing? Also, remember that all runners were new to the sport at some point, so they can all relate to the struggles that beginners face.

If you're worried about what non-runners think, try not to get too hung up on that. Just remind yourself of all the great benefits that you're getting from running and they're missing out on. And anyone whose opinion you care about (close friends and family members) are no doubt impressed and inspired that you're doing something to improve your health and fitness. Be proud!

**Dress like a runner.** As just discussed in this chapter, wearing the right clothes for running may make you feel more comfortable when running in public. You don't need to go out and buy five new running outfits, but a comfortable pair of running shorts or pants and a sharp-looking running shirt, paired with the right running shoes, can really give you a confidence AND motivation boost. Feeling good about yourself when you run will serve as a reward for your runs, which will reinforce your running habit.

**Run like a runner.** You may also feel more confident about running if you're using proper running form. See the running form tips in the next chapter to learn how to look comfortable and feel at ease while you're running. Even if your form isn't perfect, you'll feel better knowing that you're working on it.

**Run with others.** You may also feel less self-conscious if you get a friend or family member to come along with you. An added bonus to running with a buddy is that you can keep each other motivated to run. You could also look for a local running group. Check with your gym, local running store, or your town or city's recreation department to see if there are any programs for beginner runners.

**Just get moving.** Like anything else, the first time is usually the hardest. Once you've run in public a few times, you'll feel a lot more confident and comfortable, and be less concerned about others watching you.

# Chapter 4
# Tips for Proper Running Form

*"There isn't anything that isn't made easier through constant familiarly and training. Through training, we can change. We can transform ourselves."*
-Dalai Lama

Discomfort while running is a big reason why some runners get discouraged and may give up on the sport. Yet discomfort can often be remedied with some minor tweaks to your running form. Improved running form can also prevent future injuries, which will keep you running longer and stronger. You'll also run much more efficiently if you use proper running form. Follow these tips to work on developing the correct running form.

**Keep your feet pointed straight ahead.** Make sure your toes are pointed in the direction you want to go. Running with your feet pointed in or out for long stretches could lead to running injuries. If your feet naturally point outward or inward, focus on running with your toes pointing straight ahead for short stretches. The more you practice it, the more natural it will feel.

**Look up and ahead.** Keep your eyes focused on the ground about 10 to 20 feet ahead of you. Some runners are tempted to look down at their feet. Don't do it! If you're staring at your feet, you're more likely to hunch over, which can lead to neck or shoulder pain. Looking ahead is also a safer way to run because you'll be able to notice potholes, bumps in the sidewalk, sticks and other hazards and avoid falling.

**Don't overstride.** Some new runners tend to reach out to take longer strides and end up overstriding, which wastes energy and can lead to injury. To avoid overstriding, try to focus on your feet landing directly beneath your hips.

**Focus on taking short, quick steps.** Keep your stride low to the ground and focus on quick stride turnover. Try to avoid bouncing and bringing your knees up high. You'll waste a lot of energy, pound your joints and fatigue your muscles if you have too much up-and-down movement. Keep your feet close to ground, but don't drag them. You should be taking short, light steps, as if you're stepping on hot coals. Don't try to lengthen your stride or reach forward with your foot.

**Rotate your arms from the shoulder.** Swing your arms back and forth from your shoulder joint, not your elbow joint. Think of your arm as a pendulum, swinging back and forth at your shoulder. Focus on driving your elbow backwards and then let it swing back toward you. You should almost feel your hand grazing your hip as your arm rotates forward. If you're having a hard time getting the swing right, practice it while you're speed walking first, then transition into a run.

**Keep your hands at your waist.** Try to keep your hands at waist level, right about where they might lightly brush your hip. Your arms should be at a 90 degree angle. Some beginners have a tendency to hold their hands way up by their chest, especially as they get tired, and start to look like a T-Rex. You may actually get even more tired by holding your arms that way and you'll start to feel tightness and tension in your shoulders and neck. You'll also lose the momentum and power that you get from rotating your arms at your shoulders.

**Run tall.** Make sure your posture is straight and erect. Keep your head up, your back straight, and shoulders level. Don't lean forward or back at your waist, which some runners do as they get fatigued. Imagine yourself as a puppet with a string on top of your head that's pulling you upright.

**Keep checking your posture as you're running.** Your shoulders should be relaxed and square or facing forward, not hunched over. Keep your shoulders under your ears and maintain a neutral pelvis. When you're tired at the end of your run, it's common to slump over a little, which can lead to neck, shoulder and lower-back pain. Stick your chest out when you feel yourself slouching over. This also opens up your lungs more, so it'll be much easier to breathe.

**Keep your arms at your sides.** Avoid side-to-side arm swinging. If your arms cross over your chest, you're more likely to slouch, which means you're not breathing efficiently. Inefficient or shallow breathing can also lead to side stitches, or cramps in your abdominal area. Imagine a vertical line splitting your body in half – your hands should not cross it.

**Keep your hands in a loose fist.** Try to keep your arms and hands as relaxed as possible. You can gently cup your hands, as if you're holding an egg (or a potato chip, if you prefer) and you don't want to break it. Don't clench your fists because that tightness will move up your arms, shoulders and neck.

## When Will Running Start to Feel Easier?

When they first get started with running, many beginner runners have a hard time getting adjusted to their new form of exercise. Since new runners struggle for different reasons, there isn't a "one-size-fits-all" answer to the question, "When does running get easier?" Of course, one of my favorite answers to that is, "It doesn't get easier, you just get stronger." But a lot of new runners do say that things feel a little easier and more comfortable once they were able to run continuously for 30 minutes. For most new runners, that milestone can take anywhere from two to eight weeks, depending on your starting point.

So, if running even for just five minutes at a time feels like a struggle for you, stick with it and try to be patient as you continue to build up your endurance and fitness. You'll get there! In the meantime, here are some ways to help make running easier.

**Run at a conversational pace.** As a beginner runner, you should do your runs at an easy, conversational pace, which means that you can talk comfortably (in full sentences) with someone as you're running. If you're running by yourself, a good way to know you're running at a conversational pace is if you're able to comfortably sing a short song such as "Happy Birthday." If you can't do that and you feel yourself gasping for air, slow down or take a walk break.

**Check your breathing.** Another way to make sure that you're not running too fast is to make sure you're not out of breath. If you feel yourself huffing and puffing during the run, slow down and take deep breaths – from your belly, not your chest.

**Set mini-goals.** Choosing short-term goals to work toward can also help with the mental challenges of running longer. Your goals can be as simple as running to the next mailbox or lamp post. Once you reach it, pick a new target. It may feel like a lame goal but, who cares? As long as it keeps you going, it's serving its purpose.

**Beat boredom.** Some beginner runners are fit enough to run a certain distance, but they have a hard time pushing past boredom or other mental challenges during their runs. In many cases, it's simply "mind over matter." Try to distract yourself by playing mind games, choosing new running routes or running with a group. Treadmill running is perfect for catching up on your favorite shows or listening to music or audiobooks.

# Chapter 5
# Treadmill Running Tips

*"Dear Treadmill, I hate you…but I need you. Relationships are complicated."*
-eCards

Over the years, I've had a love/hate relationship with my treadmill, but I've come to appreciate the benefits of treadmill running. It's a great alternative when weather or safety issues make it impossible to run outside. And I love that I can do a very exact, targeted workout on the treadmill and know my pace, distance and hill incline for every second of my run. Follow these tips to make your treadmill running more effective, enjoyable and safe.

**Don't skip your warm-up.** Before getting started with your run, run or walk at a slow, easy pace for 5 to 10 minutes.

**Use a slight incline.** Set the treadmill incline to 1% to 2%. Since there's no wind resistance indoors, a gentle uphill better simulates outdoor running. Of course, if you're just getting started with running, it's OK to keep it at 0% as you're building up your fitness.

**Don't make it too steep.** At the same time, don't set the incline too steep (more than 7%) – this may lead to Achilles tendon or calf injuries. Also, don't run at an incline of more than 2% for the entire duration of your run. If you want to run hills, make sure you're also incorporating some intervals at 0% or 1%.

**Don't hold onto the handrail or console.** Some people assume that they should be holding onto the handrails when walking or running on a treadmill. The handrails are only there to help you safely get onto and off of the treadmill. When running on the treadmill, use good upper body form by keeping your arms at your sides, at a 90-degree angle, just as you would if you were running outside.

**Don't lean forward.** Make sure to keep your body upright. It's not necessary to lean forward because the treadmill pulls your feet backward. You need to pick your feet up from the treadmill before they are driven away by the belt.

**Don't forget your cooldown.** If you just hop off the treadmill once your workout is done, your heart rate will be elevated. Spend five minutes doing a slow jog or walk at the end of your run and allow your heart rate to go below 100 bpm before you get off. Cooling down will help prevent dizziness or the feeling that you're still moving when you step off the treadmill.

# Chapter 6
# 30-Day Beginner Running Program

*"Allow yourself to be a beginner. No one starts out being excellent."*
-Unknown

Now that you've got some of the basics about running, it's time to get started. While some brand-new runners may want to start with a simple, small habit like running for five minutes a day, others who are already active may want to follow a beginner running program. Following a schedule will help kick-start your running habit because you'll know exactly what you need to do each day and you can check off each day as you go along. This program features very gradual increases in running so you'll ease into it and won't get discouraged.

This schedule is the perfect way for a new runner to build up their endurance and start forming a running habit. To begin, you only need to be able to run for one minute at a time. Using a run/walk method, which alternates between intervals of running and intervals of walking, you'll work your way up to running continuously for 20 minutes in 30 days.

In the next chapters, we'll talk about how to make this running habit stick and how to overcome any potential obstacles and setbacks along the way.

**Week 1:**
- **Day 1:** After a 5-minute warm-up with a brisk walk, begin your run/walk intervals. Run at an easy pace for 1 minute, then walk for 5 minutes. Repeat that sequence 3 times. For your walk portions, make sure you're not taking a leisurely stroll. You should pump your arms, so that your heart rate stays elevated. That way, you'll still be getting a

good cardiovascular workout and it will make your transition back to running intervals so much easier.

- **Day 2:** After a 5-minute warm-up with a brisk walk, run at an easy pace for 1 minute, then walk for 4 minutes. Repeat that sequence 3 times. Try to work on using proper running form.
- **Day 3:** Rest
- **Day 4:** Do a 5-minute warm-up with a brisk walk, then run at an easy pace for 2 minutes, then walk for 4 minutes. Repeat that sequence 3 times. Try to work on proper deep belly breathing to help avoid side stitches.
- **Day 5:** Rest or cross-train (activity other than running). If you don't feel like taking a complete rest day today, you can do 30 to 45 minutes of a low-impact cross-training activity, such as swimming, walking, elliptical trainer, cycling, rowing, Pilates, yoga and strength-training. Those types of cross-training days are considered to be rest days because they give the joints and muscles you use in running a break, reducing your risk of injury.
- **Day 6:** After a 5-minute warm-up with a brisk walk, run at an easy pace for 3 minutes, then walk for 3 minutes. Repeat that sequence 3 times.
- **Day 7:** Rest

**Week 2:**

This week you're going to continue increasing the amount of time you're running and decrease your walking intervals.

Here are your workouts for this week:

- **Day 8:** After a 5-minute warm-up with a brisk walk, run at an easy pace for 4 minutes, then walk for 2 minutes. Repeat that sequence 3 times.
- **Day 9:** Rest or cross-train
- **Day 10:** After a 5-minute warm-up with a brisk walk, run at an easy pace for 5 minutes, then walk for 2 minutes. Repeat that sequence 3 times.

- **Day 11:** After a 5-minute warm-up with a brisk walk, run at an easy pace for 6 minutes, then walk for 2 minutes. Repeat that sequence 3 times.
- **Day 12:** Rest
- **Day 13:** After a 5-minute warm-up with a brisk walk, run at an easy pace for 7 minutes, then walk for 2 minutes, then run at an easy pace for 7 minutes.
- **Day 14:** Rest or cross-train

**Week 3:**

Running should feel a little bit easier this week. If you're still struggling, don't worry – you'll start seeing improvements very soon, as long as your maintain your consistency.

Here are your workouts for this week:
- **Day 15:** After a 5-minute warm-up with a brisk walk, run at an easy pace for 8 minutes, then walk for 2 minutes. Repeat that sequence twice.
- **Day 16:** Rest
- **Day 17:** After a 5-minute warm-up with a brisk walk, run at an easy pace for 10 minutes, then walk for 2 minutes. Repeat that sequence twice.
- **Day 18:** Rest or cross-train.
- **Day 19:** After a 5-minute warm-up with a brisk walk, run at an easy pace for 12 minutes, then walk for 2 minutes, then run at an easy pace for 6 minutes.
- **Day 20:** After a 5-minute warm-up with a brisk walk, run at an easy pace for 13 minutes, then walk for 2 minutes, then run at an easy pace for 5 minutes.
- **Day 21:** Rest

**Week 4:**

You now have three weeks of running under your belt, and you should be feeling really good about your progress. This week you're going to keep making small increases in your running intervals.

Here are your workouts for this week:

- **Day 22:** After a 5-minute warm-up with a brisk walk, run at an easy pace for 14 minutes, then walk for 2 minutes, then run at an easy pace for 5 minutes.
- **Day 23:** Rest or cross-train.
- **Day 24:** Warm-up with a 5-minute brisk walk, then run at an easy pace for 15 minutes. Then walk for 2 minutes, and run at an easy pace for 4 minutes.
- **Day 25:** Rest.
- **Day 26:** After a 5-minute warm-up with a brisk walk, run at an easy pace for 16 minutes, then walk for 1 minute, then run at an easy pace for 4 minutes.
- **Day 27:** Rest or cross-train.
- **Day 28:** After a 5-minute warm-up with a brisk walk, run at an easy pace for 18 minutes, then walk for 1 minute, then run at an easy pace for 3 minutes.
- **Day 29:** Rest.
- **Day 30:** Congratulations on making it to Day 30! Try walking for 5 minutes to begin and end the workout (your warm-up and cooldown), and run for 20 minutes in between.

**PART TWO**

# MAKE YOUR HABIT STICK

*"If you believe you can change – if you make it a habit – the change becomes real."*
-Charles Duhigg, *The Power of Habit*

# Chapter 7
# Create a Habit Loop

*"Motivation is what gets you started. Habit is what keeps you going."*
-Jim Ryun, first high school athlete to run a sub-4:00 mile

Right now you may be feeling motivated to start running. But what you'll soon realize, as Jim Ryun said in the above quote, is that motivation is not enough. At some point, your motivation will fade, you get busy with work and life, and running slips to the bottom of your to-do list. You may have already experienced this pattern with running, or some other healthy habit you wanted to adopt. We all have those items on our New Year's resolutions lists that seem to re-appear every year.

In their book, *The Power of Full Engagement*, authors Jim Loehr and Tony Schwartz write about the difficulties of making lasting change in our lives:

> "Change is difficult. We are creatures of habit. The problem with most change is that conscious change can't be sustained over the long haul. Will and discipline are far more limited resources than most of us realize. If you have to think about something each time you do it, the likelihood is that you won't keep doing it for very long. The status quo has a magnetic pull on us."

If you want to run regularly, or do anything on a regular basis, you need to make it a habit, something that you do almost automatically. You may be wondering: But is it really possible for running to become a habit? Like brushing your teeth? The answer is absolutely YES, but it helps to first understand how habits form.

In his book, *The Power of Habit: Why We Do What We Do in Life and Business*, author Charles Duhigg explains how habits shape our lives and how we have the power to shape our habits. He describes the process of habit formation as a three-step loop:

> "First, there is a cue, a trigger that tells your brain to go into automatic mode and which habit to use. Then there is the routine, which can be physical or mental or emotional. Finally, there is a reward, which helps your brain figure out if this particular loop is worth remembering for the future. Over time, this loop – cue, routine, reward; cue, routine, reward – becomes more and more automatic. The cue and reward become intertwined until a powerful sense of anticipation and craving emerges."

So how can we use this habit loop of cue, routine, reward to create a running habit?

## Why Cues Are Important

The most consistent exercisers are ones who create a habit that was triggered by a cue, according to a 2016 study in the journal *Health Psychology*. The cue, which can be something as simple as your alarm going off in the morning, triggers an automatic response to go to the gym, get dressed for a run or do some other exercise-related routine. The routine is something that you don't even have to deliberate – it's just an automatic decision instigated by your own internal or environmental cue.

In the study, researchers compared this type of habit, known as an instigation habit, with an execution habit, which is having a plan for a specific type of exercise. They wanted to find out which type of habit would help people stick with an exercise routine over the long-term.

At the start and finish of the month-long study, they asked 123 university students and faculty questions to determine how often they exercised and how strong their exercise habits were – whether they did it without thinking, for example. From these questions, the researchers gleaned whether a person had a strong instigation habit or a strong execution habit.

They discovered that the only factor that predicted how often a person exercised over the long-term was the strength of their instigation habit. Researchers also found that the strength of the instigation habit increased with the frequency of exercise, whereas the execution habit didn't really change in relation to frequency. So the more you use a cue to trigger your runs, the more ingrained your running habit will become.

## Choosing Running Cues

So, since cues can help you be more consistent with exercise, what sort of cues will help trigger a running routine? Some people use cues without even realizing it, or perhaps they use a different cue on different days of the week, depending on when and where they're running. If you run in the morning three times a week, you may use an alarm clock cue. For your evening runs, your cue may be walking through your door after work. Below are some more ideas.

## For a morning running habit:

- Hang your running schedule in a prominent place, like on your refrigerator, so you see it every day.
- Put your running shoes by your bed.
- Leave your running shoes by the door.
- Lay out your running clothes on your floor.
- Leave your phone and headphones on your dresser.
- Place a light, pre-run breakfast, like a banana and a yogurt, on the kitchen counter.
- Wake up to a motivating song on your alarm, so you'll get pumped for your run.
- Tape a note with your distance goal on your bathroom mirror.

- Leave your water bottle on the kitchen counter.
- Place your running watch next to your bathroom sink.
- If you have a pet, tie your running habit to a pet chore (i.e., go run after feeding the dog).
- If you drink coffee before running, leave your running watch by the coffee maker.

**For an evening running habit:**
- Put a reminder on your phone to signal when it's time for your run.
- Change into your running clothes as soon as you get home from work. Lay them out before you leave for work in the morning, so they're ready for you when you get home.
- Put your running shoes by your front door so you see them when you arrive home.

**For a (home) treadmill running habit:**
- Place your phone (or other listening device) and headphones on the treadmill.
- Put your running shoes on the treadmill.
- Place your water bottle on the treadmill.

**TO DO: Plan your running cues.**

Using this list or your own ideas, come up with some running cues that work best for your schedule and situation. You may decide to add some additional ones along the way, but it's important to establish some triggers for your running routine.

While you're planning your running cues, pay attention to other cues that may be inhibiting your running habit. Do you hit the snooze button instead of getting up to run? Do you head right to the pantry or fridge when you get home from work?

Once you're more aware of the "bad habit" cues, you can more easily change the behavior. Strategize ways to avoid those cues and substitute your new running cues. Place your alarm clock across the room, so you're not tempted to snooze. Change into your running clothes as soon as you get home from work so you go for a run instead of snacking or plopping down on the sofa.

## The Power of Rewards

Linking your running routine to an external reward is the final step of the neurological habit loop. "An extrinsic reward is so powerful because your brain can latch on to it and make the link that the behavior is worthwhile. It tells our brain whether we should store this habit for future use or not," Duhigg explains. "It increases the odds the routine becomes a habit."

In addition to their role in the habit loop formation, rewards can just make life more fun and interesting. In her book, *Better Than Before: Mastering the Habits of our Everyday Lives*, habits and happiness expert Gretchen Rubin says that giving ourselves rewards can boost habit formation. "When we give ourselves treats we feel energized, cared for, and content, which boosts our self-command – and self-command helps us maintain our healthy habits," she writes. "Studies show that people who get a little treat in the form of receiving a surprise gift or watching a funny video, gained in self-control." Rubin explains that if you deny yourself treats you'll start to feel depleted, resentful, justified in self-indulgence and more likely to break your good habits.

Studies have confirmed the power of rewards in creating an exercise habit. Researchers at New Mexico State University interviewed 266 people who exercised at least three times a week to determine why they were able to consistently exercise over the long term. In one group, 92 percent of people responded that they continued to exercise because it made them "feel good." In another group, 67 percent of people said that exercising gave them a feeling of "accomplishment."

For new runners, it may take some time to experience the "runner's high" – that good feeling that occurs at the end of a run when your body releases feel-good endorphins and neurochemicals. And they may not immediately feel the satisfaction of checking off a workout after it's done and measuring their progress. Duhigg writes:

> "But countless studies have shown that a cue and a reward, on their own, aren't enough for a new habit to last. Only when your brain starts expecting the reward – craving the endorphins or sense of accomplishment – will it become automatic to lace up your jogging shoes each morning. The cue, in addition to triggering a routine, must also trigger a craving for the reward to come."

I've been running since I was a kid, so it's hard for me to remember a time when I didn't know what it meant to feel a runner's high, or that feeling of satisfaction after completing a long or difficult run. But I can easily understand how those post-run good feelings might not be automatic. It helps to think about it in terms of other types of exercise, or basically anything that is difficult the first few, or many, times you do it. My (dreadful) experience with hot yoga comes to mind.

My friend Christina loves yoga, especially hot yoga classes. Although I'm not a big yoga person myself, I was intensely curious about hot yoga, and she convinced me to join her in a class. I told her I was extremely nervous and she confidently shook her head, "You run marathons, you'll be fine. Bring two bottles of water. And two towels." Gulp. Was I really ready for this if I was already intimidated just hearing the packing list?

We were only about 20 minutes into the 90-minute class when I was already regretting my decision. I was completely drenched, my face was beet red and I felt like I was standing on lava. Yet everyone else in the room was calmly and gracefully executing the moves, as if there was a giant fan oscillating in front of us. Christina, cool as a cucumber, was flawless and looked like she could easily fill in for the instructor at a moment's notice.

*Why was I the only one constantly glancing back at the door? Would anyone notice if I tried to make a run for it?* So many questions were running through my head. Two in particular that kept popping up were, *Why would anyone in their right mind want to subject themselves to this kind of torture? And pay for it?*

Two wet towels and a couple of giant water bottles later, I made it through the 90 minutes, thanks to some breaks in the "rest" position.

I was grateful that I survived, swore to myself, "Never again," and then was incredulous to see so many smiling faces and satisfied looks as we walked out of Dante's Inferno back into room temperature.

I found Christina and wanted to bow down before her, in awe of her mental and physical strength.

"You're amazing," I said to her. "That was one of the hardest things I've ever done. How do you do it? Why?!"

"Oh, you get used to the heat," she said. "I just love how I feel afterwards. I did it. I made it through."

Suddenly it clicked. Christina was getting the same endorphin-releasing, mood-boosting reward that I get after completing a long run or finishing a race. After taking the class many times and getting used to the extreme heat, Christina now craved the reward of feeling accomplished for getting through an incredibly tough class. Although I saw hot yoga as a torturous activity that I couldn't wait to end, if I stuck with it, I might too start craving that reward.

When a behavior becomes habitual, our brain strongly associates certain cues with certain rewards. Soon your brain will start craving that reward. Until then, you can help force certain behaviors, such as running, to become a habit by consciously setting rewards for it. In the case of the hot yoga class, I didn't experience the accomplishment reward, as my friend did. So if I wanted to continue with hot yoga, I'd have to consciously set some extrinsic rewards (an iced coffee in air conditioning, perhaps?) to get the habit going, until the intrinsic rewards of achievement and pride started kicking in.

## **Choosing Rewards**

As is the case with many running-related things, your miles may vary. A reward that works for one runner may not work for another.

One reward I've had great success with over the past two years is listening to audiobooks while running. It may not be for everyone and it's actually something that I resisted for years when some running friends encouraged me to try it. ("But doesn't listening to a book instead of reading it feel like cheating?" I'd say.)

But I tried it once and became hooked. Using the Hoopla app on my iPhone, I download free audiobooks, anything from juicy novels to biographies to parenting advice books. While this reward may not work for everyone, I find myself craving the next chapter and looking forward to my runs more than ever before. I actually start thinking of my long runs in terms of how many chapters I'll be able to get through in my book.

In the past, I always had trouble finding the time to read, but now I find myself averaging a book every 10 days or so. Seeing how quickly I got through my first book helped me immediately let go of my hang-up about "cheating" by listening. Here I was actually finishing a book in a week, rather than picking it up intermittently over the course of a couple of months.

I keep a list of books I've read so far this year and I add a new one each time I finish it. Watching that list grow over the year makes me feel accomplished for not only finishing the books, but also for running all the miles while listening to them. And, a sidenote: Maintaining a "books I've read" list is also helpful when I want to recommend a book I've read to a friend and, for the life of me, can't remember the title. A funny quirk about listening to audiobooks is that you're not always looking at the book's cover, title and author, so it's easy to forget the exact names.

What I've discovered is that I have a couple of rewards associated with listening to audiobooks while running. I have the immediate reward of listening to a book that I'm interested in, but I also have a longer-term reward of feeling accomplished and satisfied for reading more books. I feel like I successfully mutli-task reading and running. An additional and quite unexpected reward is that many of the books I've read have led to fun and interesting conversations with friends and family members.

To be sure, listening to audiobooks (or podcasts, if you prefer) may not work as a reward for everyone. But to get your own running habit rolling, you'll need to find a few rewards that will motivate you.

In terms of daily (or almost daily) rewards, it's important to keep them small and not too indulgent, to avoid developing unhealthy habits while trying to retain or establish good ones. If your reward for every run you do is a chocolate-covered donut, you could negate many of your run's benefits and find yourself on a slippery slope toward more unhealthy habits. Before you know it, you're washing down the donut with a caramel-topped latte and eating fast food for lunch, convincing yourself it's a suitable reward for your morning run.

Below is a list of healthy rewards for runners that you might use to complete that habit loop of cue, routine, reward. Although not all may work for you, pick some out and add your own ideas.

## Short-term Reward Ideas for Runners
- Hot bubble or sea salts bath
- Watch a favorite show while running on the treadmill
- Listening to music while running
- Iced or hot coffee
- Playing with a dog or cat
- Cup of tea
- Downloading some new songs for your playlists
- Run to meet a friend for coffee
- Taking a nap
- Hot shower
- Playing a game with a kid
- Watching a game on TV

- Researching races to run
- Using an app on your phone that gives you rewards for exercise, like CharityMiles, which tracks your mileage and allows you to earn money for charities when you run or walk
- Reading running quotes
- Running at a totally new and beautiful location (like near water)
- Running with a friend to catch up
- Foam rolling session
- Reading a gossip magazine
- Watching some funny videos on You-Tube
- Being lazy on the couch
- Recording your run details in your training journal, schedule, or app
- Drinking a healthy smoothie after a long run
- Playing a game on your phone
- Checking social media
- Checking off a completed workout on your calendar
- Putting a dollar in a jar after each run and treat yourself when you reach a goal

## Longer-term Reward Ideas for Runners

- Manicure or pedicure
- Massage
- New running gear, like a visor, running shorts or socks
- Going out to dinner to celebrate finishing a big race

## TO DO: Make your list of running rewards.

Write a list of ideas for rewards and keep it in your training journal or somewhere prominent, like on your calendar or training schedule, so you're frequently reminded of your motivations. Plan out some rewards. You may want to choose some immediate rewards for each run you complete and longer-term rewards for when you reach a particular milestone.

You'll probably need different rewards for different types of runs, depending on when or where you're running. For instance, your treadmill run reward may be binge-watching your favorite show, while an outdoor run may end at your favorite coffee shop to meet a friend.

As you're planning your runs for the week, make sure you think about your rewards. It helps if the reward is tied into the routine itself, like listening to your favorite playlist while running. Delayed rewards aren't always as effective as immediate ones.

As your runs develop into a habit, your rewards will become more intrinsic – such as a feeling of satisfaction or pure joy from having completed a run. But, as you're getting started and trying to establish your running habit, you should also use extrinsic rewards to start creating that habit loop.

# Chapter 8
# State Your Plans

*"If you run, you are a runner. It doesn't matter how fast or how far. It doesn't matter if today is your first day or if you've been running for twenty years. There is no test to pass, no license to earn, no membership card to get. You just run."*
-John Bingham, running writer

### Habit-Making Strategy: Call Yourself a Runner

If you ask 10 different people what it means to be a runner, you'll get 10 different answers. When does a person cross that line between being a casual jogger and a runner?

Dr. George Sheehan, a best-selling author from the 1970s running boom, is quoted as saying that "the difference between a runner and a jogger is a signature on a race application." Of course, that quote is little dated, since most people now enter races online with no signature required, but you get the idea. Basically, if you've been doing it for long enough that you entered your first road race, you're a runner – regardless of when you started running or how fast you are.

I'd argue that participating in a race shouldn't be a requirement to call yourself a runner. I know plenty of people who have been running for years but have never put on a race bib and run from a starting line to a finish line. I've also talked to runners who have run races who've said that they still don't consider themselves a runner. They'll explain by saying that they think of runners as people who run really fast or have been running for many years.

The term runner for some people may be uncomfortable because, even though they run, they don't actually like running (yet, I would argue!). I can understand that better if I relate it to something that I do but don't really enjoy. For example, I'll go fishing with my dad, but I can't say I enjoy it (the fishing part) and I definitely wouldn't call myself a fisherwoman. My goal is to spend some quality time with my dad, doing something he enjoys.

So, I suppose that to be a runner you have to run on a regular basis and enjoy running (most of the time, anyway). Beyond that, there really isn't any strict definition or standard for what constitutes "running." When you decide to call yourself a runner is a matter of personal preference. There's no required time period, pace test, or mileage threshold you need to pass. Runners are of all ages and shapes and sizes, so you're never too young, old, big or small to be a runner. Some people will call themselves a "fitness jogger" or "someone who runs" rather than identifying themselves as a "runner." Sometimes it takes hearing someone else call them a runner (as in, "This is my friend, Camille. She's a runner.") for them to actually consider themselves one.

"We are what we repeatedly do," according to Aristotle. My advice is to embrace being a runner. Once you start to call yourself a runner and see that as part of your identity, you'll begin to embrace running as more of a part of your life — not just some fleeting interest. Your running habit becomes an extension of who you are, so it's a lot harder to break.

## Habit-Making Strategy: Tell Others

Start sharing your desire to start a running habit with family and friends. By telling others, you'll be making yourself more accountable. Knowing that your friends and family members will be asking you for updates about your progress will help you stay motivated to keep running.

Your desire to start a running habit will also feel much more real once you start telling people. Think about this in terms of other habits you've tried to start in the past. If you kept your goal to eat more fruits and vegetables to yourself, you wouldn't feel much pressure about your food choices when eating with friends. But if you tell some friends, family members or co-workers that you're going to eat a lot healthier, you'll probably choose much healthier options when they're around. Telling others gives you a lot more accountability. If you choose not to tell people about your goal of establishing a running habit, you have to honestly ask yourself, "Is this something that I really want to do?"

Also, your friends and family members may have some good advice and offer much-needed moral support and encouragement. You may want to post occasional updates on Facebook or other social media to share your progress and stay accountable. Notice how I said share "occasional" updates. Don't be an over-sharer! If you post about every detail of all your runs, you'll risk annoying your friends, who may stop encouraging or asking about your new running habit.

When you tell friends and family members about your plans, you may be surprised to hear them say that they too want to start a running habit. You can plan to do some runs or maybe even a race together or, at the very least, check in on each other about your progress. Having an "accountability buddy," with whom you can check in with about your running progress, is highly recommended. You're more likely to stick to your running schedule when you know you have to report to someone else about it.

## TO DO: Tell at least one person about your new running habit.

If you've already told someone, tell another person. Make sure it's someone you know will be supportive and encouraging. Keep them updated about your progress.

## Habit-Making Strategy: Ask for Advice

Seeking the advice of an expert is one of the most valuable yet underused aspects of habit formation. Chances are you know some other runners, so why not ask them for advice? Runners love to talk about running. If you start asking a runner questions, you may actually find that you have a hard time getting him or her to shut up.

Even if the runner isn't a seasoned veteran, that's OK. You don't have to get answers to really technical questions. But you may want to ask for tips on where to shop for shoes, good places to run, how to avoid painful chafing and how they felt when they were first getting started. All runners are different, but hearing various perspectives on running may just lead you to certain strategies and tips that will work for you. If you're struggling, you'll be relieved to hear from other runners that they too had a hard time when they first started running. Talking to others about running may also help you find some new running buddies and start building a running network. At the very least, you'll get some encouragement and motivation.

## TO DO: Ask another runner for tips.

Tell a runner you know that you're getting started with running and want to ask their advice. More than likely, they'll be flattered that someone is seeking their opinion about running. If you don't know any other runners or just don't feel comfortable asking for advice in person, go virtual. Post your questions on running blogs, online running forums or Facebook pages for *Runner's World* or other big running websites or groups. You're sure to get some helpful responses and you may find yourself a supportive virtual running community.

# Chapter 9

# Plan Your Runs

*"If you fail to plan, you are planning to fail."*
-Ben Franklin

Beyond the habit cycle of cue, routine, reward, there are other behaviors and strategies you can employ to reinforce your running habit and help you maintain focus and motivation. They can reinforce and nurture a new habit and help it grow into a strong habit that's tough to break.

A big key to habit formation success is to plan, plan, plan. Like most things that we'd like to do, if you don't plan out when, where and how you're going to run, it's probably not going to happen. So to get your running habit moving forward, you need to start making some solid plans.

## Habit-Making Strategy: Make Running a Priority

Some people say that they can't find the time to run or do other forms of exercises. They're right, actually. Most people aren't going to suddenly find a block of free time, hidden in between juggling a full-time job, making meals and doing errands.

Even if you do manage to find some spare minutes, if running isn't a priority, you're going to fill that time with checking social media, watching TV or some other activity that feels more fun than running. To start a running habit, you need to MAKE time for running, rather than just expect that time to magically appear.

One way to figure out when you can find time to run is to track everything you're doing in a typical week. Maybe there are some things you're doing that you're willing to cut out in order to make more time for running.

Everyone's priorities are different, so it's up to you to decide what you can live without. I like to keep a clean house, but I definitely enjoy running much more than cleaning. So I'm willing to sacrifice a perfectly spotless and tidy house. Scrubbing the floors can wait – I need to go for a run.

So, in addition to saying you want to make running (and good health) a priority, you also need to figure out what things are NOT as important. For instance, it's OK to say no to the laundry, the gourmet meals made from scratch, the pointless work meetings and the unanswered emails. Let go of the guilt. Track your time over a week and look for opportunities to avoid wasted time and squeeze in more running time. You may find out that you're spending several hours a week plopped on the couch watching televison. Or you may discover that you're doing a lot of chores or tasks that you could farm out to other family members or pay someone else to do.

Look for ways to fit running into your schedule. Why not DVR your favorite shows so you could watch them a lot faster and use the extra time for a run? Or, run on a treadmill or do another workout while watching your favorite shows. If you spend a lot of time shuttling your kids back and forth to activities, see if you can arrange a carpool with other parents to save time. Or, try doing a run in between drop-off and pick-up instead of wasting time driving back and forth from home. An added bonus is that you'll get to discover some different running routes.

According to time management expert and author Laura Vanderkam, when we say we don't have time for something, what we're really saying is that it's not a priority. In researching her book, *I Know How She Does It: How Successful Women Make the Most of Their Time*, Vanderkam asked extremely busy women to compile a time diary, in which they track their time for a week, recording how they spent every hour of every day.

In her TED talk, "How to Gain Control of Your Free Time," Vanderkam explains how a busy working mom in one of these time diary studies came home to find that her water heater was broken. Cleaning up the immediate mess and dealing with the aftermath (having a plumber come to replace the water heater, getting the carpets cleaned) took up seven hours of her week.

Vanderkam says:

> "But I'm sure if you had asked her at the start of the week, 'Could you find seven hours to train for a triathlon?' 'Could you find seven hours to mentor seven worthy people?' I'm sure she would've said what most of us would've said, which is, 'No – can't you see how busy I am?' Yet when she had to find seven hours because there is water all over her basement, she found seven hours. And what this shows us is that time is highly elastic. We cannot make more time, but time will stretch to accommodate what we choose to put into it…we have the power to fill our lives with the things that deserve to be there."

Vanderkam recommends writing down some goals and the steps you need to take to achieve them:

"Maybe you want to run a 5K. So you need to find a race and sign up, figure out a training plan and dig those shoes out of the back of the closet. And then – this is key – we treat our priorities as the equivalent of that broken water heater, by putting them into our schedules first. We do this by thinking through our weeks before we are in them."

And that brings us to our next strategy.

## Habit-Making Strategy: Plan Your Runs Out on Sundays

At the beginning of the week (Sunday is always a good day for planning it out), look at your calendar and make time for running. As much as possible, try to stick to a consistent schedule from week to week. You don't have to run at the same time every day you run, but if you start setting a regular running schedule, you're more likely to get in the habit of running and stick with it.

By determining when, where, and how your runs will happen, you don't have to think much about getting it done. Research has shown that this type of specificity does help people stick with a new habit. In one study about exercise compliance, a group of non-exercising college students were given data about how exercise could significantly reduce their risk of coronary heart disease. Participation in the fitness group increased from 29 to 39 percent. However, when the students received the heart disease information and were also required to indicate when and where they planned to exercise, compliance went up to 91 percent.

Other studies regarding healthy eating habits have found similar results. Study participants were much more likely to eat healthy, low-calorie foods when they were asked in advance to say what they planned to eat for each meal.

When plotting out your running plan for the week, think carefully about your schedule, existing habits and temperament to determine what will work best for you. Some runners run in the morning and there are numerous benefits to morning running, as discussed later in this chapter. But you should plan your runs for when they work best for you. I know lots of runners who prefer to run in the evening after work, as a way to unwind and recover from a long, stressful day. Going for a run before heading home is a way to create a transition between work and home.

You may want to consider some other factors when planning out your runs. I always plan my weekly running schedule on Sunday while looking at the weather forecast on weather.com. I plan my longest runs of the week on the days when the weather is looking most favorable. If I know it's going to be a torrential downpour or bitterly cold, I make that a treadmill (shorter run!) day.

This strategy doesn't always work out perfectly – sometimes my schedule isn't that flexible. I've certainly done my fair share of runs in the rain or the freezing cold when I already had an outdoor run planned with my team or I just couldn't bring myself to do a long run on the treadmill. But I find that consulting the weather forecast makes me more likely to get my runs done since I probably won't use bad weather as an excuse to not run.

It also helps if you make plans with a running buddy, so you're both held accountable. It's a lot harder to blow off a 6:00 a.m. run when you know your friend is waiting for you. And if you keep a regular running date, everyone in your life is more prepared to deal with it. So, for instance, the kids know that running with your friend on Wednesday nights or your running group on Saturday mornings is just part of mom's or dad's routine.

## **TO DO: Plan a week of runs.**

Whether you want to plan to run five minutes a day, use the 30-Day Beginner Schedule in the previous section or one of the schedules in the back of this book, or come up with your own plan, schedule the runs that you'll do for this coming week. Put them on your paper calendar, in your phone calendar, in a training journal or on a sheet of paper that you hang on the fridge. Just make sure you'll see them written down somewhere. Having your runs planned out someplace other than just your head will increase your chances of actually doing them.

After your first two weeks of regular runs, analyze what days and times have worked best for your schedule and routines. How did you feel after running in the morning? Are you an evening runner? What days of the week worked best for you to run? Take note of what worked and what didn't as you're making your plans for next week.

### **Habit-Making Strategy: Remind Yourself**

When I schedule my weekly runs, or any other exercise plans, in my phone calendar, I always set reminders. If I want to do a boot camp class at my gym, I need to sign-up for the class the day before, so I put a reminder in my phone to do that and then another reminder for the class itself. Many days I don't forget that I have a run or other exercise planned, but there are some days when I'm completely spacing out or stressed and I really need the reminder.

Setting reminders is especially critical during the first few weeks of habit formation when the reminder can serve as one of your cues (in our cue, routine, reward loop) to start your run.

## Habit-Making Strategy: Run on Mondays

If you belong to a gym, you may have noticed that it's a lot harder to get a treadmill on Mondays, compared to other days. And it makes sense. Let's face it: Mondays are tough. Starting the week out with an endorphin-boosting run or other workout can make us ready to face and help us deal with the anxiety, stress and fatigue that Mondays can sometimes bring.

I try to run every Monday and I always feel like I'm starting off my week on the right foot. It's motivating and satisfying to check something off my to-do list so early in the week. It's like getting a head start on the week. Feeling that sense of accomplishment gives me a boost of motivation and confidence that gets me through the week and inspires me to get some more runs in. And that reward will force a running habit into a deeper groove.

Another benefit of running on Monday is that a last-minute invitation to blow off your run and do something else is less likely to pop up on a Monday. Think about it: Who is going to try to cajole you into going to Happy Hour on Monday night? Not much is happening on Monday evenings, so it's a good time to go for a run outside or hit the gym. Or, if you wake up early to do a run Monday morning, you're not going to feel like you're missing out on much if you're tired and hit the hay early Monday night.

To understand the effectiveness of running on Mondays, it helps to think about how you might feel when you don't start your week out with a run. If you give into the pressures of work or family commitments or the desire to sleep in a little, you're more likely to continue that pattern. Similar to the feeling of falling off track on a diet, you might think, "Well, I'm already off schedule this week" and be less motivated to stick to your plan for the rest of the week.

Running on Monday sets a solid pattern for the rest of the week.

**TO DO: Plan to run on Mondays.**

When planning your runs for the week, make sure you schedule some miles on Monday. The reward of feeling accomplished (and hopefully less stressed) will reinforce your commitment to complete your other scheduled runs for the week. Once you've run for several Mondays in a row, you'll start to crave those rewards and you'll be well on your way to establishing a Monday running habit.

Here are some tips to make sure you get in a Monday run:

**Put it on your calendar.** This is the number one reason I'm successful at getting my Monday runs done. I block out time, even if it's just a half-hour, and I treat it just like an appointment that I need to keep.

**Prep for it.** To guarantee yourself a Monday run, you need to prep for it in advance. Lay out your running clothes and gear on Sunday night, when you have a little more time to get organized, so you're ready to go on Monday.

**Plan a reward.** As I already mentioned, Mondays can be tough! Give yourself a little reward for starting out the week right with a run. Plan for a post-run coffee or other mini-treat to give yourself something to look forward to.

### Habit-Making Strategy: Make Your Progress Visible

Seeing a record of your progress can be extremely powerful. Mark your runs and other workouts on a calendar and check them off as you go along. Seeing all those accumulating checks or X's will give you a tangible, visible reminder of your progress and serve as motivation to maintain your running habit.

Some runners keep a training log or a running blog to track their progress. Jot your workout in your notebook and write some notes after each one. Be sure to mark the date, your approximate mileage and time, and a few comments about how you felt (i.e., "finished strong," "felt sluggish first 2 miles.")

Keep your log in a prominent place to help remind you (and maybe put a little pressure on you) to keep running. Or, if you prefer to do it online, create a running blog and post entries about your progress and share it with friends and family.

There are lots of great running apps, like RunKeeper, that help you keep track of your runs on your phone. You may want to use a social fitness-tracking app, like Strava, so you can track your runs and also get the benefits of a supportive network of other runners. A recent study in *Nature Communications* actually found that using a social fitness-tracking app may actually help motivate you to run longer and faster. Researchers found that if one person ran for about 10 minutes more than usual on any given day, their Strava friends would increase their workouts by approximately three minutes, even if the weather conditions weren't ideal. They also found that if a friend ran faster than usual, his or her friends would tend to pick up the pace in their runs that same day.

Another benefit of tracking your workouts is that you know what you've done in the past, so you can try to improve your workouts to get fitter and stronger. Most of us do not have photographic memories and won't remember what runs we did last week, let alone last month. Having a digital or paper record of what you did will allow you to see how far you've come and how to challenge yourself in your upcoming workout.

To get stronger and fitter, you need to continually challenge yourself to up the intensity of your workout. Without tracking how hard you worked in the previous week's sessions, you won't know how much to push yourself in your current workouts. If you did three sets of ten push-ups last week, you should be trying for three sets of twelve push-ups this week.

## TO DO: Make a plan to track your workouts.

Whether it's a wall calendar with your planned runs jotted down, a notebook used as a training journal, a printed training schedule or a running app on your phone, figure out how you want to keep track of your runs. As you continue to check off your workouts, you'll look forward to the reward of checking off another run and get motivated by seeing all those workouts recorded.

## Habit-Making Strategy: Run in the Morning

*"Running is kind of like coffee. The first time you drink it you might not like it. It's bitter and leaves a bad taste in your mouth but you kind of like the way it makes you feel. However, after a few times, it starts to taste better and then all of a sudden you're hooked and it's the new best part of waking up."*
–Amy Hastings Cragg, U.S. Olympic marathoner

How you start your day often sets the tone for the rest of the day, and running in the morning always makes me feel like I'm starting out my day on the right foot. I feel more energized, alert, productive and in a good mood. It's a relief to not have the pressure of squeezing in a run at the end of the day and I always feel like I've gained some extra time in the day.

Research has actually shown that runners who run in the morning are more consistent with their running than those who try to do it in the afternoon or evening. For most people, mornings are the most predictable and least demanding part of the day, so you're more likely to stick to your plan. Evening exercise plans are often derailed by work or family obligations or just pure exhaustion at the end of the day. It's much easier to blow off your run after you've worked all day and just want to collapse and be a lazy lump on the couch.

Our willpower gets tested and sometimes used up throughout the day, so it can be tough to muster the self-discipline to run after a long day at work. If you plan to wake up a little bit earlier and run in the morning, your willpower tank is full. But our willpower is a limited resource. If you have a tough day at work and you burn through a lot of your willpower by staying on task and keeping yourself from blowing up at annoying co-workers, you may have very little willpower left by the time you get home. It might be easy to blow off your run. But if you get your run done in the morning, you'll be taking advantage of your full willpower reserves and you'll avoid giving into laziness later in the day. An added bonus is that you'll feel more energetic and be more productive during the day. You may even have a little more patience to deal with those, um, irritating colleagues.

Morning runs are also good preparation and training for races, since most are run in the morning. If you typically run in the morning, your body will already be used to the routine on race day. I always like to tell runners that I coach, "Nothing new on race day," so you shouldn't be running in the morning for the first time on the day of your race.

Running in the morning can also help with weight loss efforts. A morning run will jump-start your metabolism, so your body burns calories at a faster rate during the day. You'll also feel tired at night and go to bed earlier, thereby reducing the number of hours when you're tempted to snack late at night.

I remember seeing a quote once that said, "Run in the morning before your brain figures out what you're doing." It's meant to be funny, but there's also some truth to it. During our morning routines, we do so many things that are habitual – get up, make coffee, eat breakfast, shower, get dressed, brush teeth. We don't even have to think about these things. If you can incorporate a run into your morning, it becomes part of your routine.

As mentioned in the discussion about habit cues, there are many different cues you can use to trigger a morning run habit. It may be unrealistic to try to run or exercise every morning, but if you aim for two or three mornings a week, you can establish a solid morning running habit. Here are some tips to get your morning running habit going:

**Get to bed early.** A morning running habit starts with proper planning the night before. Some people think they can watch late-night TV and still get up early for a run. Do yourself a favor – DVR your favorite late TV shows and plan to get to bed in time to guarantee yourself 7 to 8 hours of sleep. Once you've done a couple of morning runs, you'll start to get more tired at night, so it will be easier to get to bed early.

**Sleep in your running clothes.** This trick may seem a little silly, but I know plenty of runners who have tried it and say that it works.

**Or, lay out your clothes.** If you don't feel like sleeping in your clothes, at least lay them out, all ready to go. That will be your cue for your morning run. And having your clothes right there will make it easier to get dressed to run. Check out the weather forecast so you're prepared for the conditions. You won't be able to blow off your run because you couldn't find a specific pair of shorts or piece of gear. And you'll start getting dressed for your run before you even have a chance to consider not doing it. Some runners even like to put their clothes in the bathroom, which forces them to wake up a little and then get dressed. (Added bonus: If you have a snoozing partner next to you, he or she will appreciate not being disturbed.)

**Put your alarm clock out of reach.** When that alarm goes off early in the morning, it's tempting to keep hitting the snooze button and skip your running plans. But if your alarm clock is across the room, you're already out of bed and a lot less likely to say, "Just 10 more minutes..."

**Follow a training schedule.** If you're training for a specific race and following a training schedule, it's much harder to blow off those morning runs. You'll think to yourself, "I have to be ready for that half-marathon," or, "My schedule says 5 miles today. Gotta run." Even if you're not training for a specific race, you can write your planned runs on your calendar at the start of the week. Then, stick to the plan.

**Think about your plan the night before.** Plan out your morning run the night before – how far, for how long and what course you'll run. Doing so will help you get more motivated for your run and ensure that you have enough time to run before you start the rest of your day.

**Get a morning running buddy.** If you usually run by yourself, try to recruit a running friend to meet you in the morning. Or, find a running group that meets in the morning. You'll be less likely to skip your run if you know people are waiting for you.

**Eat something light.** It's never good to run on an empty stomach, but you most likely won't have a lot of extra time to eat and then digest your food. Try eating something small like an energy bar or a banana, so you're not running on empty. Make sure you also drink some water when you wake up, so you're hydrated for your run.

## Habit-making Strategy: Don't Think All or Nothing

Even if you start with just a 5-minute daily run, you'll eventually want to expand to longer runs and have a regular running schedule. But that doesn't mean that there won't be days when it may be impossible to stick to your exact schedule. On those days, don't assume that you shouldn't run at all if you can't do what you originally planned. If you start skipping runs completely, you may slide down a slippery slope. One missed run turns into two skipped runs and so on. Rather than skipping the entire run, do what you can. Run for a mile or two, if that's all you have time for. One mile is better than no miles, and going through your running routine, regardless of the distance you run, will help deepen the groove of your habit.

Beyond the habit-building benefits, you'll also make some fitness and health gains with shorter runs. Frequent, shorter runs help your body adapt better than infrequent longer runs. You're also less likely to get injured if you run consistently, as opposed to taking the "weekend warrior" approach of cramming lots of exercise in on the weekends. So you're actually better off doing three 20-minute runs during a week than just one hour-long run. That brings us to our next habit-making strategy – the mini habit.

## Habit-making Strategy: Start with a Mini Habit

Much research has been done and books written about the benefits of starting mini habits, also sometimes called tiny habits or micro-habits. In his book, *Mini Habits: Smaller Habits, Bigger Results*, Stephen

Guise explains how starting with a very small daily habit, such as one push-up a day, can lead to big results. How exactly? Once you start a mini running habit, even if it's running for a minute or two each day, you begin the habit formation process and work on strengthening your self-discipline and willpower. As the habit takes hold and your willpower improves, you can build on that habit, adding more time to your runs.

Establishing a running habit with the mini habits approach can help you avoid a pattern that may be familiar to you: Aim for a big goal, take a few steps toward it, lose willpower and momentum, quit, feel like a failure. When people take on too many changes at once, they can overwhelm their limited supplies of willpower and discipline. Most often, they simply give up. "The result is not just that you failed to stick to your plan, but that you also likely fed your belief that it's impossible to change lifelong habits," write Jim Loehr and Tony Schwartz in *The Power of Full Engagement*.

With a mini habit, the opposite scenario plays out. You're consistently completing your goal, so you'll feel positive and encouraged to keep going. You start to see progress, so you begin to believe that, yes, it's possible to create a new, healthy habit.

When I first heard about the concept of mini habits, I was intrigued. Since I've been running for years, I didn't need to start a running mini habit, but there were plenty of other healthy habits or productivity improvements I wanted to implement. I had been wanting to try meditation for a while, after hearing a lot about its benefits from books, articles, and friends. I always felt I didn't have the time. But surely I could spend one minute a day meditating, right? I started that a couple of months ago, and now I'm up to a 10-minute meditation every weekday afternoon. I'm already noticing that I feel more calm after meditating, and now I've started to crave that reward.

The key to making the mini habit approach work is to pick a goal that's "too small to fail." So commit to running for just five minutes every day. Each time you do your mini running habit, you'll also be taking steps as part of your routine, such as changing into your running clothes, putting on your running shoes and cueing up your running music. All of these steps will become cues that signal the start of your running routine.

## Chapter 10
## Practice Healthy Habits

*"Take care of your body. It's the only place you have to live."*
-Jim Rohn, motivational speaker and author

When I'm extremely busy, I find that some of my healthy habits, such as healthy eating and getting plenty of sleep, go right out the window. My poor nutrition and lack of sleep lead to low energy, which makes it much harder to get motivated to run.

On the other hand, when I make sure I get plenty of sleep and focus on eating healthy, I'm more energized and inspired to run. Healthy habits are contagious. If I'm rested and fueling properly, my runs feel better and that encourages me to keep my running habit going. But if I let some of my healthy habits slide, it becomes much easier to let my running habit also slip away.

### The Importance of Sleep

"I'm too tired" is a frequent excuse for not exercising. And it makes sense. When we don't get enough sleep, our willpower is weakened and we're more likely to overact to stress and give into unhealthy temptations.

But lack of sleep doesn't just affect your willpower and energy levels. In her book, *Thrive: The Third Metric to Redefining Success and Creating a Life of Well-Being, Wisdom, and Wonder*, author Arianna Huffington stresses the importance of sleep for living a full life and adhering to other positive, healthy habits. "Sleep deprivation reduces our emotional intelligence, self-regard, assertiveness, sense of independence, empathy toward others, the quality of our interpersonal relationships, positive thinking, and impulse control," she writes.

Sleep is important for anyone trying to live a healthy lifestyle, but it's especially important to runners because of the demands that we put on our bodies. Successful runners get plenty of sleep so their bodies can recover and they feel refreshed and energized for their next run. Getting to bed earlier may even inspire you to run in the morning, rather than later in the day.

### Better Sleep Tips

Aim for seven to eight quality hours of sleep a night – the right amount for most adults. If you're way off from the goal with your current amount of sleep, try to increase your sleep time in small increments. Aim for 20 minutes more a night one week, and then keep adding ten more minutes each week until you reach the recommended amount. If 20 minutes earlier feels like too much, try going to bed five minutes earlier (think mini habit!) each night. Add five more minutes the following week and so on, and soon you'll be getting the recommended amount. Once you start noticing the rewards of improved energy, increased productivity, and better mood, you'll be even more motivated to get to bed on time.

If you have trouble falling asleep, follow some of these tips:

• Avoid caffeine after 2:00 p.m., so there's time for the effects to wear off. Stay hydrated with water instead of having coffee, tea or soda in the afternoon.

• Try not to run too close to bedtime. Although regular exercise will help you sleep better, it's ideal to complete your workout at least a few hours before you hit the hay.

• While you shouldn't go to bed hungry, you should avoid eating a heavy meal before bedtime. Digesting all that food may keep you awake. Try to finish eating two to three hours before you go to bed.

• Avoid alcohol right before bedtime. Although you may think a glass of wine will help you fall asleep faster, alcohol interferes with deep sleep and increases sleep arousals, so you won't get a restful night's sleep. If you want to drink alcohol, finish it a few hours before you go to sleep so your body has time to metabolize it.

• Make sure your bedroom is comfortable and conducive to sleep.

Create a room that is dark, quiet, comfortable and cool for the best sleep possible. Evaluate if anything in your bedroom is no longer comfortable and needs replacing. Pillows should be replaced every two to three years and most mattresses are good for 10 years.

• Establish a relaxing bedtime routine, such as taking a warm bath, sipping some decaf tea, reading a book or listening to soothing music.

• Try not to watch TV or be staring at your phone or computer right before trying to fall asleep. If you have a hard time resisting your phone alerts, set it to go into silent mode an hour before bedtime. Use a real alarm clock, not your phone, so you're not tempted to check it when it's on your nightstand.

## Eat Well, Run Well

Runners need to eat healthy to fuel their workouts properly and help build stronger bodies. Try to eat a balanced, healthy diet and have your health care professional check for any nutritional deficiencies. An iron deficiency, for example, can wreak havoc on runners' training because it can lead to feelings of sluggishness and low energy. Here are some sensible and healthful eating rules to get the most out of your food – and your runs.

**1. Fill at least half of your plate with fruits and vegetables.** Vegetables and fruits are packed with nutrients that will benefit your overall health and help fuel your runs. Different vegetables and fruits supply different nutrients, so it's important that you eat a variety of fruits and vegetables. A good rule of thumb is to eat a mix of different colored fruits and vegetables. Choose red, orange and dark green vegetables such as red peppers, sweet potatoes and broccoli.

**2. Include whole grains.** Aim to make at least half your grains whole grains. Look for the words "100% whole grain" or "100% whole wheat" on the food label. Whole grains provide more nutrients, like fiber, than refined grains.

**3. Don't forget the dairy.** A cup of fat-free or low-fat milk with your meal is a great way to get your dairy requirements. You'll get the same amount of calcium and other essential nutrients as whole milk but fewer calories. Don't drink milk? Try a soy beverage (soymilk) as your drink or include low-fat yogurt in your meal or snack.

**4. Add lean protein.** Runners focus so much on consuming their carbs that they sometimes don't get the protein they need. But protein is crucial for runners, as it's used for some energy and to repair damaged tissue, such as muscles. Protein should make up about 15% of your daily intake. Runners, especially those training for long distances such as marathons, should consume .5 to .75 grams of protein per pound of body weight.

Choose protein foods such as lean beef and pork, chicken, or turkey, and eggs, nuts, beans or tofu. Try to eat seafood, such as shrimp or fish, as your protein twice a week. Beans, such as lentils, black-eyed peas, lima beans, great northern beans and chickpeas, are an easy protein to add to any meal. Try to choose entrees that feature beans, such as tacos, chili, bean soup and bean salads.

**5. Keep healthy foods close and convenient.** Try to stock your fridge and pantry with foods that make up a nutritious, heart-healthy diet, such as whole grains, fish, lean meats, vegetables and fruits. Keep cleaned baby carrots, celery sticks and other cut-up vegetables in your refrigerator so you can grab them when you want a quick snack.

**6. Eat small meals throughout the day.** Don't assume you have to eat the standard three meals a day, with a few hours in between. Runners get hungry, so that doesn't usually work for them. It's better to spread your calories out with a small meal every three to four hours. You'll find that eating mini meals will help maintain your energy levels throughout the day and keep you from feeling hungry all the time. Spreading out your calories will also help with weight loss and maintenance efforts, since you'll reduce your risk of binging when you're suddenly starving and want to eat everything in sight.

**7. Avoid extra fat.** Using heavy gravies or sauces will add fat and calories to otherwise healthy choices. Instead of heaping on melted cheddar cheese on steamed broccoli, just sprinkle it with low-fat parmesan cheese or a squeeze of lemon.

**8. Try new foods.** Keep it interesting by picking out new foods you've never tried before, like mango, lentils, quinoa, kale or sardines. Exchange fun and tasty recipes with friends or find them online.

**9. Take your time when eating.** Savor your food. Eat slowly, enjoy the tastes and textures, and pay attention to how you feel. Be mindful. Eating very quickly may cause you to eat too much, especially when you're feeling hungry.

**10. Get creative in the kitchen.** Whether you're making soup, a lasagna, or a stir-fry, find ways to make them healthier. Try using less meat and cheese, which can be higher in saturated fat and sodium, and adding in more veggies that add new flavors and textures to your meals. When you make pasta with a red spaghetti sauce, throw in onions, mushrooms and peppers. If you're making a sandwich, use whole-grain bread and lots of fixings – lettuce, tomatoes, thinly-sliced cucumbers and sprouts – to add more nutrients and fiber to fill you up. Make your own pizza and load it up with lots of veggies. Avoid getting in the habit of eating the same foods day after day. Pasta often becomes a staple of a runner's diet, but there are lots of other healthful and interesting carb choices for runners, such as couscous, rice or quinoa.

**11. Use smaller dishes.** Eating your food from smaller plates or bowls will help with portion control because you'll be less likely to take big portions. You'll feel satisfied that you finished your plate, but you'll avoid overeating.

**12. Don't deny yourself the foods you love.** If you always avoid foods you love, one day you'll have a monster craving and end up going overboard. To prevent that, you should allow yourself small portions of your favorite foods. In the long run, you'll save calories, because you'll feel more satisfied and you'll be less likely to binge and eat mindlessly. Eating in moderation is the key.

**13. Take control of your food.** Eat at home more often so you know exactly what you're eating and how it's prepared. Bring a healthy lunch to work so you're not tempted to grab fast food because you're short on time. Be prepared with healthy snacks, like fruit, plain popcorn or trail mix, at work so you don't head to the vending machine for a sugar fix.

If you eat out, check and compare the nutrition information. Many restaurants now highlight the healthiest items on their menus. Choose options that are baked (not fried) and lower in calories, saturated fat and sodium.

**14. Satisfy your sweet tooth in a healthy way.** Indulge in a naturally-sweet dessert dish – fruit! Serve a fresh fruit salad or a fruit parfait made with yogurt. Strawberries topped with fat-free Cool Whip are a delicious, low-cal sweet treat. For a warm, comforting dessert, try baked apples topped with cinnamon.

## Track Your Healthy Habits

Running often becomes a keystone habit, or a habit that causes a chain reaction of good habits and has the power to be life-transforming. Many running friends and runners whom I coach attest to the domino effect of their running habit. Brad was actually a smoker when he first started running and he found that the more he ran, the less he smoked. Other runners have told me that regular running has motivated them to establish better eating habits, drink less alcohol and get more sleep.

In some cases, running somewhat forces another healthy habit. For instance, runners often improve their sleep habits because the increased physical activity makes them need the restorative power of sleep. Or, in Brad's case, smoking made running more difficult, so he had some incentive to give it up. But, in some instances, there may not really be an impetus to start another healthy habit. Running just has a contagious effect.

So, as you continue with your running habit, you're bound to notice some positive changes in your health and body. Becoming more aware of these changes and actually measuring them will help you stay motivated to keep up your running habit.

Try to weigh yourself and take your measurements regularly (once a week is fine) so you can see your progress. Get your blood pressure and cholesterol checked and follow up to get it tested again in a few months. Take your resting heart rate every morning – as you improve your fitness, you should see it go down.

## TO DO: Choose a tiny, healthy habit to implement.

Pick one tiny, healthy habit that you can start, whether it's flossing one tooth, going to bed five minutes earlier, or eating one strawberry every morning. Start small. If possible, incorporate your new, healthy habit into your running habit routine, like drinking some water right before you start your run. Tying two healthy habits together like that increases your chances of success.

## Chapter 11
## Run With a Group

*"Running is not, as it so often seems, only about what you did in your last race or about how many miles you ran last week. It is, in a much more important way, about community, about appreciating all the miles run by other runners, too."*
-Richard O'Brien, British actor

Running with others is one of the most effective strategies for running habit formation and maintenance. Indeed, the social benefits of running are among the biggest reasons why runners start and stick with running. Whether you're running with one friend or a large running team, here are some ways runners can benefit from being part of a group:

**You'll have built-in role models.** People naturally start to adopt habits of those around them. Spending time with other runners will help immensely with your habit formation because you'll start to mirror your running friends' habits.

**You'll motivate each other.** With a running group, you get a built-in cheering squad. Members cheer for each other at races and support one another during long runs. You'll be more motivated to stick to your training because you'll hold each other accountable. It's harder to blow off a workout when you know others are expecting you to be there.

**You'll feel a sense of purpose.** Mentoring other runners or being part of a cohesive team can you give a sense of purpose and help you make new and meaningful connections.

**You'll get creative stimulation.** It's fun to brainstorm ideas when running with a group. You can bounce ideas off your running friends and ask them for advice.

**Your performance will improve.** Everyone thrives on a little healthy competition. When you're running with others who are pushing you to run faster and harder, it's easier to take it to the next level. When running alone, you may be tempted to cut your workout short, but peer pressure will get you to do the entire workout, and maybe even a little extra.

**You can network.** Running with co-workers, clients – even your boss – is a great way to network and build your professional relationships in an unassuming way. You'll develop a camaraderie with other runners that's difficult to replicate in an office or other work setting. Building or reinforcing relationships through running may lead to a new job or other opportunities. I know lots of runners who've made important professional connections or formed stronger bonds with co-workers through running.

**It's much safer to run with others.** Potential attackers or harassers are not likely to go after a group. It's tough to get lost if you're with a group and, even if you do take a wrong turn, you have each other to figure out how to find your way. And if someone in the group gets injured or sick, there's always someone there to help.

**You can beat boredom.** Although I do sometimes like my alone time when running on my own, my group runs fly by much faster. It's tough to get bored when you're running with others. You're also more likely to explore new running routes when running with a group, which will definitely make your runs more interesting.

**You'll feel a sense of community.** Whether you're racing together, volunteering at a race or cheering on teammates, it's fun and rewarding to be connected with like-minded people and be part of something that's bigger than you. Runners can really relate to each other and are supportive of one another through the ups and downs. Runners feel certain emotions and find humor in things that only fellow runners can understand. These bonds make runners feel like they're part of a special, tight-knit community.

**You'll expand your social circle.** Running with a group is a great opportunity to meet people with similar interests. Many people (myself included) have met their spouse, significant other or close friends through a running group or club.

## The Power of Community

One of the most compelling examples of the power of community in facilitating habit change is Alcoholics Anonymous. An estimated 2.1 million people seek help from AA each year, and as many as 10 million alcoholics have achieved sobriety from the group. The AA program is built on a system of meetings and companionship. AA insists that alcoholics attend "ninety meetings in ninety days" and each member is given a "sponsor," someone they can reach out to if they're feeling tempted to drink. The group dynamic helps AA members believe that they can make a permanent behavior change.

In *The Power of Habit*, Charles Duhigg discusses the power of AA in helping alcoholics adapt new habits and believe that they can cope with the stresses of life without consuming alcohol. Duhigg interviewed Lee Ann Kaskutas, a senior scientist at the Alcohol Research Group, who said:

> "At some point, people in AA look around the room and think, if it worked for that guy, I guess it can work for me. There's something really powerful about groups and shared experiences. People might be skeptical about their ability to change if they're by themselves, but a group will convince them to spend disbelief. A community creates belief."

I've witnessed this power of community among runners I've trained for half and full marathons. Many of them start their training declaring, "I'm not a runner. I don't think I can do this!" But then they begin to run with the group and they meet others in the same position. They find that many of the other runners are also feeling not really sure if they can take on the challenge of a long distance race.

They also meet more experienced runners in the group, and find out that they had once had been newbie runners, but they followed the training and crossed the finish line. After talking to these other runners and running alongside them, the new runners start to believe that they could rise to the challenge. They develop faith in themselves and the process, and it keeps them moving forward to their goal.

## How to Find a Running Group or Running Buddies

Not sure how to go about finding a running groups or partners? Here are some ideas to try.

**Find a local running club.** Check out the Road Runners Club of America's website (www.rrca.org) to find the club closest to you. Many running clubs' websites have forums or databases where members can post requests for running buddies. You can scan through the posts and see if someone matches your pace and schedule. You can also go to their group runs to find runners at your level and pace.

**Check with your local running store.** If you're lucky enough to have a local running store, take advantage of this incredible resource. Many running stores offer group training runs, usually for free, that start and finish at the store. Even if they don't host runs, the employees are part of the running community and can probably suggest local running groups to you. They may also have postings on their bulletin board from people looking for running partners.

**Ask at your gym or health club.** Check your gym's bulletin board for notices or sign-ups for running clubs or running partners. Or, ask a staff member if they know of any trainers or gym members who lead running groups. If your gym doesn't offer anything like that, ask if it's OK if you post a note saying that you're looking for a running buddy. Because other gym members are likely to have similar fitness goals, chances are good that you'll find someone.

**Find a charity group training program.** Many non-profit organizations offer coaching and cover race expenses in exchange for your fundraising efforts. You'll get training guidance and motivation by running with others training for similar races.

**Volunteer at a road race.** While you're sitting at the registration table or handing out water at an aid station, you'll probably meet other runners who are looking for running partners or know about local running groups.

**Register for a local race.** Many races offer free group training runs to registered participants. If you're training for a specific race, check the race website to see if they have any organized training runs scheduled. Even if they don't offer organized training runs, you may meet some new running buddies during or after the race.

**Recruit runners at work.** Ask around at work and see if anyone would be up for running before work, during lunch or after work. See if you can rally the troops to register for a local race. Training for and running a race together could be a great bonding and team-building experience and you may get to know fellow employees who you may not otherwise have met.

## How to Start a Running Group

Finding the right running club or team can sometimes feel like dating. But, unlike the search for a perfect mate, if there's a dearth of running clubs in your area or you haven't found one you like, you could always create your own. Here's what to do:

**1. Start with a few core members.** To get a club going, you really need two or three committed people. Recruit one or two running friends or co-workers and pick a race that you can train for together.

**2. Get the word out.** Go beyond the "word-of-mouth" approach by posting flyers at running and athletic gear shops, gyms or other places where active people might be. If you want to get the group started at a specific place, like work or school, ask if you can do an email blast or post on the organization's website. Use Twitter and Facebook to spread the word to your virtual friends.

**3. Plan your runs.** To get the best attendance, it's good to start with an informal Saturday or Sunday run of three to six miles. As the group gets bigger, you could add another short run or speed work during the week and have two weekend runs – a short one and a long one for those training for longer distance events. Ask other members to lead the runs so they can contribute to the group.

**4. Make new members feel welcome.** Give special attention and get to know new members so they don't feel like it's a cliquey running group. Try to match them up with another runner at their pace and running ability so they have someone to run with.

**5. Plan social events outside of the runs.** Running clubs don't have to be just about running! Schedule post-run brunches, holiday parties or BBQs. Social outings help people meet other club members they might not run with and give them another reason to keep showing up for runs.

## Chapter 12

## Train for a Race

*"So much in life seems inflexible and unchangeable, and part of the joy of running and especially racing is the realization that improvement and progress can be achieved."*
-Nancy Anderson, running coach

Training for a race is one of the most effective ways for runners to keep running. The pressure of having a deadline – race day – will motivate you to make sure you find time to run. Registering for a race and paying for your race entry in advance also makes you feel more dedicated to your running, since you've made a financial commitment and have some "skin in the game."

And the motivational power of racing is enduring. Once new runners cross that first finish line, the huge rush and the reward of the accomplishment they feel propels them to their next race. So many of the runners I've coached have become "hooked" after experiencing the magic of their first race.

In the back of this book, I've included beginner schedules for 5K (3.1 miles), 10K (6.2 miles), half marathon (13.1 miles) and marathon (26.2 miles), which are the most common race distances.

You may be tempted to start with an ambitious goal, such as a half marathon, but I recommend that beginners begin with a 5K race. You should be able to find a local 5K fairly easily. You can always move up from there! Many local and national non-profit organizations organize 5K races as fundraisers. Check websites such as Active.com to search for races in your area.

Once you've found a race, here's some basic advice for your training and race day. If you're not quite ready to race, be sure to come back and check these tips when the time is right.

## Training Tips

**Stick to the schedule.** Following a training schedule will not only keep you motivated, but it will also help prevent you from getting injured by doing too much too soon. If you feel like you could do more than the schedule calls for, do some cross training. Strength-training, especially your core and lower body, is extremely beneficial to runners. You can train with light weights, take a boot camp and strengthening class, or do some simple bodyweight exercises. Other excellent cross-training activities for runners include cycling, swimming, water jogging, yoga and Pilates.

**Practice running outside.** It's fine to do some of your training on the treadmill, but make sure that you also do some runs on roads. You use different muscles when you run outdoors so, if you only run on a treadmill, running outside may feel harder. Doing some of your miles outside will help get you more physically and mentally prepared for the race. If you're doing a local race and have access to the course map (check the race website), try running part of the course during your training so you're a little familiar with it. Doing so will give you a big confidence boost because you'll have an idea of what to expect.

**Run with others.** Training and racing is more fun if you do it with a friend or family member. You can also help keep each other on track and motivated. Even if you don't run with a friend or a running group, try to run where other runners or walkers will be, such as the park, the local high school track or running trails or paths. Being around other runners will boost your motivation to keep running. You may even end up finding some new running partners.

**Don't run like crazy the week before.** You're not going to get any fitter or faster in the week before your race, so don't try to cram for the final. Do three easy runs of 25 to 30 minutes during the week. Some people like to rest the day before the race, while others like to do a 10 to 20-minute shake-out run to help them stay loose. It's up to you to decide if you want to rest or do a shake-out run, since there's no evidence that one strategy is better than the other.

## Racing Tips

The days and morning before a race can be filled with anxiety, even if you've raced before. Here are some tips to help you feel more race-ready and confident.

**Get your race outfit ready.** Check the weather forecast and plan your race outfit accordingly. Lay everything out the night before, so that you're not rushing around in the morning and more likely to forget something. You should race in clothes that you've run in before, so you don't have any unexpected discomfort or issues like chafing. Nothing new on race day!

If you have the opportunity to pick up your race bib the day before the race, do it. You'll be able to pin your bib on (to the front, not the back, of your shirt) at home and not be rushing to pick up your number before the race.

**Don't start out too fast.** One of the biggest rookie race mistakes is to start at a fast pace, only to totally lose steam in the final mile. Don't worry about the runners sprinting past you in the beginning. Start at a pace that you know you can hold for the entire race distance.

**Don't fear the water stops.** Some new runners get nervous about dealing with water stops in the race. You may see some runners cruise through, grab a cup and drink the water, but you don't have to do it that way. It's not necessary to keep running through the water stop. Some race participants will walk through so that they can carefully take the cup from the race volunteer and sip it, without spilling the water or having to gulp it down. If the race conditions are very cool, some 5K racers find that they don't even need water and they opt to skip the water stop. Other runners carry their own water bottle so that they can drink some water when they need it.

**It's OK to walk.** Some beginner runners worry about having to take a walk break during a race because they think they'll look or feel like a failure. They equate walking with giving up. There's no shame in taking a walking break! You may actually find them to be beneficial. Some race participants find that taking short walk breaks actually helps them achieve an overall faster race pace than if they tried to run the entire distance.

**Finish strong.** As you get closer to the finish line, there's no holding back – if you feel good, go for it. Keep pumping your arms and looking ahead. Try to "go fishing" and catch some runners in front of you. Imagine you're reeling them in and see if you can pass them before the finish line.

**Use a mantra.** Pick a short phase, such as, "Just keep moving," "One step at a time" or "Strong or steady!" that you play over and over in your head while running. Repeating a mantra can help you stay focused and be your inner motivation when you need it most. Mantras can be especially helpful when you're struggling towards the end of a race and you keep repeating, "I can do this" or "I am tough", to push yourself to the finish line. (For some running mantra suggestions, go to run-for-good.com/the-power-of-mantras.)

## How to Deal With Pre-Race Nerves

Race anxiety can be an obstacle for some runners, especially beginners. But there are strategies to manage pre-race nerves and actually make them work to your advantage. Here are some ways you can deal with performance anxiety, take advantage of your pre-race excitement, and make racing a fun and motivating aspect of your running:

**Practice deep breathing.** If you're anxious, your breathing becomes shallow. Breathing deeply from your belly has a calming effect and it can also prevent side stitches. Work on belly breathing during your training runs and, by race day, you'll do it without even having to think about it. If you have trouble practicing deep breathing on your own, try doing a guided breathing meditation using an app such as Calm or Take a Break.

**Say, "I'm excited!"** Rather than telling yourself (and anyone else who will listen!) that you're so nervous and afraid, keep repeating, "I'm so excited!" Just calling your pre-race anxiety something positive can completely reframe it and make you see it as an encouraging, motivating force rather than a debilitating one. Your "excitement" will make you feel pumped and ready to take on your race.

**Visualize your race.** Swimmer Michael Phelps, the most decorated Olympic athlete of all-time with 28 medals, is well-known for his mental toughness and pre-race preparation. His long-time coach, Bob Bowman, designed a visualization routine for Michael when he was a young swimmer, to help him stay calm and focused. In *The Power of Habit*, Charles Duhigg describes what Phelps did when Bowman instructed him to "watch the videotape":

> "The videotape wasn't real. Rather, it was a mental visualization of the perfect race. Each night before falling asleep and each morning before waking up, Phelps would imagine himself jumping off the blocks and, in slow motion, swimming flawlessly. He would visualize his strokes, the walls of the pool, his turns, and the finish, He would imagine the wake behind his body, the water dripping off his lips as his mouth cleared the surface, what it would feel like to rip off his cap at the end. He would lie in bed with his eyes shut and watch the entire competition the smallest details, again and again, until he knew each second by heart....Eventually, all Bowman had to do before a race was whisper, 'Get the videotape ready,' and Phelps would settle down and crush the competition."

While Phelps' visualization techniques were obviously effective for him, you don't have to go to such lengths to reap the benefits. A couple of weeks before your race, begin visualizing yourself starting, running and finishing. Envision your race plan and how you'll want to feel. Think positively about your training and tell yourself that you'll feel confident and ready.

If you keep using these visualization techniques, that positive mind-set will become second nature on race day. You'll also start feeling much more positive during your training runs as well.

**Do an easy warm up.** Standing around at the starting area can make you even more nervous. Go for a five-minute jog to clear your head and stay loose. Do some dynamic stretches to get your blood flowing and muscles ready. Focus on taking deep breaths.

**Use music.** Many athletes like to listen to music as part of their pre-race ritual. Like many other Olympic athletes, Michael Phelps also used music as a pre-race ritual and calming strategy. Before every race, he'd put on his headphones, listen to the same playlist and continue the same pre-race ritual that he had been doing for years.

Create a playlist of songs that get you pumped and listen to them as you warm up or just sit and relax before heading to the starting line. Listening to the same songs for every race will be your cue to signal that it's almost "go time." In addition to helping you get in the zone, listening to music is an easy way to drown out other runners' nervous pre-race chatter.

## Curing the Post-Race Blues

*"It's important to know that at the end of the day it's not the medals you remember. What you remember is the process – what you learn about yourself by challenging yourself, the experiences you share with other people, the honesty the training demands – those are things nobody can take away from you whether you finish twelfth or you're an Olympic Champion."*
–Silken Laumann, Canadian Olympian

A first-time marathon finisher recently confessed to me that, rather than wanting to celebrate her accomplishment, she felt sad and disappointed after her race. It may sound crazy to some, but her experience is actually pretty common among runners. After spending months training and focusing on a goal, it abruptly comes to an end once they cross the finish line, leaving them feeling bummed-out, disconnected and even depressed.

No matter what distance race you're doing, even if the race went well, you may feel sad and a bit lost now that it's over. Those feelings can wreak havoc on your running habit, since you may start feeling so bummed out that you just want to stop running altogether.

Here are a few ways to cure or at least ease the pain of the post-race blues:

**Be prepared.** Even if you don't expect to get bummed-out once your race is over, it's good to be ready for it just in case. Make plans for the weeks following your race, so that you'll be distracted from that disappointed feeling.

**Keep your running habit going.** You don't have to run at the same intensity you were when you were in training mode. But don't get out of the habit of running, since not running for a week or two may make it very difficult to re-start your habit. And you may start to feel even worse once you realize that you have to work hard once again to re-establish your running habit. The post-run endorphins will help you break out of your post-race funk.

**Set new goals.** Some people start feeling disappointed because they no longer have a major goal to focus on. Your goal doesn't have to be a race of the same distance that you just ran – you may want to focus on running faster at a shorter distance, or try something completely new like a triathlon. Having another goal to focus on will help you stick to your running habit.

# PART THREE

# OVERCOMING ROADBLOCKS AND SETBACKS

*"If you're trying to achieve, there will be roadblocks. I've had them; everybody has had them. But obstacles don't have to stop you. If you run into a wall, don't turn around and give up. Figure out how to climb it, go through it or work around it."*
–Michael Jordan

## Chapter 13
## Be Prepared for Setbacks and Negative Thoughts

*"We can derive as much value from studying and understanding our failures as we can from celebrating and reinforcing our successes."*
-Jim Loehr and Tony Schwartz, The Power of Full Engagement

Even the most consistent runners face obstacles such as injury, illness, work and family responsibilities, and basic boredom. In 15 years of coaching thousands of runners, I've never coached a single runner who didn't have a lapse along the way. No one has ever done 100% of the runs or races they planned to do. Life happens. I've missed short runs, long runs, minor races and big races because of weather, injuries, boredom, exhaustion, illness, pregnancy, scheduling and just plain fear.

Slip-ups do happen, and it's important to mentally prepare yourself for them and tell yourself how you'll get back on course. In her book, *The Sweet Spot: How to Find Your Groove at Home and Work*, Dr. Christine Carter offers excellent advice for how to respond when you stumble, so you can get back on track quickly:

> "Don't get too emotional about your slip or succumb to self-criticism. Instead, forgive yourself, remind yourself that lapses are part of the process, and that feeling bad about your behavior will not increase future success. Rededicate yourself to your resolutions (now, in this instant, not tomorrow). Why do you want to make the changes that you do? How will you benefit? Do a little deep breathing and calm contemplation of your goals.

Make a plan for next time that you will face a similar challenge. What will you do differently? What have you learned from your slip?"

Expecting slip-ups to happen and being prepared for them can help us steer clear of them when they do come our way. Think about what could possibly go wrong with your running habit and plan out ways to avoid those issues when they do happen. For example, when the weather is snowy and icy where I live, it's not safe to do my usual running routes around town. Rather than forgoing my runs, I plan in advance when and where I'll run. I've had to be flexible with my training schedule and sometimes will do a long run a day or two before it was originally planned so I can get it done before a big storm hits. Or, I'll suck it up and do a treadmill run.

When you do fall off track (which will happen!), don't beat yourself up. Judging or punishing yourself isn't going to help you get back on track or avoid future falls. Rather, use it as a learning opportunity. Think hard about why and how you got off track. Is your goal too ambitious? Do you need to rethink your priorities? Are you holding on to an old habit that is making your running habit difficult to implement?

## TO-DO: Determine your challenges.

Write down the most likely challenges that you'll face as you move ahead with your running habit. If you've tried running or other forms of exercise before, what were your obstacles? Are you concerned about lack of time? Motivation? Are you worried about getting injured? Then, think about what you'll do when those problems arise. And brainstorm ways that you can anticipate those issues and avoid them being an obstacle to your progress.

In this section, I've got lots of tips for how to handle all kinds of possible setbacks and roadblocks, from lack of time and motivation to injuries and illness to unsupportive family members.

## Be Ready for Negative Thoughts

*"You have to want it, you have to plan for it, you have to fit it into a busy day, you have to be mentally tough, you have to use others to help you. The hard part isn't getting your body in shape. The hard part is getting your mind in shape."*
-Amby Burfoot, chief running officer, *Runner's World*

Sometimes it's not enough to think positive. In order to combat negative thoughts and a pessimistic attitude, it helps to anticipate them. Say what?! It may seem counterintuitive or not very motivating, at the very least, to be thinking negative thoughts before they even happen but, as is the case with many running-related things, it's always good to be prepared. Negative thoughts are going to sometimes intrude and they're part of the process – not a reason to give up. If you have specific strategies for handling your negative thoughts, they're much less likely to bring you down or throw you off your running habit.

You'll most likely have some negative thoughts or doubts regarding your running abilities. You may think, "This is so hard" or "I'm never going to be able to run faster or farther." Here are some ways to effectively deal with those types of negative statements that may pop into your head:

• **Counter them.** Have some positive statements ready to counteract these thoughts when they pop into your head. Tell yourself, "I've come so far from where I started" or "I've made so much progress." Congratulate yourself for getting started in the first place.

• **Use the word "but" to interrupt negative thoughts.** Amend your negative thoughts with a "but" statement. For example, "Running is hard for me, but if I keep doing it, it will start to feel easier."

• **Maintain your perspective.** Don't compare yourself to other runners or beat yourself up for skipping some runs here and there.

Think about how far YOU have come and how you're taking steps to improve your health with a running habit. Don't jump to conclusions and assume that a few missed runs means you've completely lost the fitness that you worked so hard to build up. Things are rarely as bad as they may initially seem.

- **Avoid all or nothing thinking.** Don't assume that a few missteps mean that you're going to fail. Avoid making broad generalizations such as, "I always fail when trying new habits" or "I'll never be a runner." Tell yourself that setbacks and roadblocks will happen, but you'll work around them and continue on your path. No one is perfect, so embrace your imperfection! And recognize that there will be some bumps along the way.

# Chapter 14
# Embrace Positivity

*"I run because it's so symbolic of life. You have to drive yourself to overcome the obstacles. You might feel that you can't. But then you find your inner strength, and realize you're capable of so much more than you thought."*
-Arthur Blank, co-founder of Home Depot

A few summers ago, I was training two women, who were longtime friends, for a marathon. They were both beginner runners, but one woman was a total Negative Nelly and kept focusing on the challenges and her own personal struggles. She'd say the training was too hard, the race was too long, the weather was terrible, and she'd never be fit enough to complete a marathon. Her friend, on the other hand, approached the race with confidence and determination, knowing that – although it wouldn't be easy – she would work hard to reach her goal.

Guess which one of them actually crossed the finish line? Let's just say that Negative Nelly was still complaining from the sidelines, never acknowledging that her negative attitude had anything to do with not being able to adequately prepare for the race.

While no one wants to be a total pessimist, a huge, intimidating goal such as running a marathon might bring some negative feelings to the surface. But if you let those feelings take control, you're almost guaranteeing yourself a bad result. For example, say I have a tough workout to do, and I start the run thinking, "This is going to be hard. I can't do this." Feeling terrible about my workout before it even starts is an excellent way to make sure that it's going to be a difficult, miserable experience. It becomes a self-fulfilling prophecy.

The way you think about a workout or race can be so powerful that it can also have the opposite effect. If you direct your thinking in a much more positive way, and tell yourself, "I can do this. I feel strong. I am strong," then you start to believe it and the workout is much more successful. Even if you do have a bad run, look for the positive by telling yourself, for example, how you're mentally tougher as a result. And getting a run done is better than no run at all.

Although positive energy is obviously not a substitute for training, your running will be much more successful if you think and stay positive, no matter what happens. And you'll be much more likely to stick to your running habit.

## Keep Your Self-talk Positive

Motivational self-talk is a tool that sports psychologists often use, and studies have found that self-talk can help athletes in a variety of situations. One Canadian study found that cyclists performed better in 95-degree weather after they practiced positive self-talk about handling hot weather. Research suggests that runners can especially benefit from self-talk during the later stage of a race, when discomfort and pain, as well as negative thoughts, set in.

But you don't have to be in racing conditions to reap the benefits of positive self-talk. Make sure you congratulate yourself or at least give yourself a mental high five after you've completed a run. Doing so can trigger the release of dopamine, a feel-good chemical messenger, which tells your brain that going for a run is an activity worth repeating.

Positive self-talk can speed up the creation of those desired intrinsic rewards that help reinforce your running habit. And rewards are more effective when they're built into your habit routine, so your self-talk is more likely to boost your habit than a delayed reward.

When coaching runners, I find the ones who talk positively about their progress and pat themselves on the back after completing runs are the ones who are the most consistent with their training. That doesn't mean you have to be a braggadocio to get the benefits of positive self-talk. It can be a dialogue that's completely in your head, telling yourself things like, "You're awesome!" or "You totally pushed yourself during that run!" If you feel negative thoughts entering, try to replace them with positive ones.

Stating your intentions and goals in a positive manner can have an incredible effect on your mindset. When we declare our intentions negatively, such as, "I won't eat too much dessert" or "I won't blow off my run tomorrow morning," they can chip away at our limited supply of willpower and discipline.

Making a positive statement such as, "I will get in my run tomorrow morning," is much more powerful and motivating than the negative version. If it feels awkward or uncomfortable forcing these kind of positive statements, simply try to avoid using the word "not" in your self-talk. Keep at it, and it will eventually start to feel more natural and instinctive.

You can also use these types of positive statements to prepare for a potential obstacle to your running habit. Rather than saying, "I won't skip my run if I get busy," you can tell yourself, "When I feel stressed, I'll go for a run. I'll feel better." With these types of affirmations, you're already preparing yourself for your reward for running, which will help reinforce your running habit.

And your positive self-talk doesn't have to be related just to your running habits. Congratulate yourself for completing the mini habits associated with your running habit. If you lay out your running clothes the night before a long run, tell yourself how well-organized and disciplined you are. Say to yourself, "Way to go, you did it!" when waking up early to get your morning run done.

Rewarding yourself with self-talk for those mini habits will make you more likely to do them, which strengthens your running habit.

## Create a Positive Environment

Do your best to infuse your life with positivity. Post positive quotes on your mirror or fridge, so you'll have daily reminders to keep your habit going. (Check out http://run-for-good.com/inspiring-running-quotes for some motivational running quotes.) Listen to positive, uplifting music, audiobooks or podcasts when you're running or doing chores around the house.

Try to surround yourself with positive people. If someone in your life is very negative and always seems to bring you down, try to limit your time with that person, especially if they're discouraging or disparaging your new interest in running.

Set up your home so that you're not always tempted with foods or activities that will distract you from or take you off course from your running and other health-related goals. For example, try to limit the amount of junk food in your kitchen, so you're not constantly feeling like you're having to resist cravings.

"If you know that you have limited willpower, that willpower is best invested in setting up a positive environment rather than waste it in having to fight against a poor environment," writes Derek Doepker in his book, *The Healthy Habit Revolution*. "Keep in mind that while you can't always get rid of negative environmental influences, such as co-workers and family members, you can usually always do something to add in more positive influences."

## TO DO: Pick three simple ways you can make your environment more positive.

Ask yourself this question: What are the top sources of negativity in my life? Whether it's specific people, certain websites or your surroundings, figure out what those negatives influences are and how you can limit your time with them. If it's not possible to reduce the impact of all three influences, then try to focus on one or two.

With the time you've saved by avoiding those influences, try focusing on three ways you can add more positivity to your life, whether it's listening to relaxing music or uplifting podcasts in your car, making a healthy meal, clearing out some clutter in your home, strengthening your relationships with supportive people or seeking out new, positive sources.

## How to Deal with Unsupportive Family Members or Friends

*"Keep away from people who try to belittle your ambitions; small people always do that – but the really great make you feel that you, too, are great."*
-Mark Twain

One obstacle to running habit formation that people tend to overlook is an unsupportive partner or other family member. Your mate's resentment or jealousy may get in the way of your running. Sometimes a partner or close friend may worry that their relationship with you is in jeopardy because of the time and attention you're giving to your new running habit. Or they may also want to also try running but are tooafraid of failure.

Talk with your partner or friend about how important running is for your physical and mental health. Have an open and honest conversation about what you both think is a fair balance between time spent training and time spent together. Good communication will help avoid future conflicts.

Be sure to spend some quality time with them so they are reassured that you're not going to become so consumed with running that you neglect your friends and family members. Schedule plans with your partner or friends the same way you plot out your runs. When they see that you're still making them a priority, they won't feel as threatened by your new running habit.

Although it may not work with everyone, another strategy is to convince your partner or friend to join you. Even if you can't get them to start running, your enthusiasm may encourage them to exercise or find a new hobby that ignites their passion. You can find a way that you can exercise together, like you running while your friend or family member is biking.

If all that fails, it may be a sign that you're dealing with a toxic relationship and you need to limit your time with that person. Life's too short to waste time on people who bring you down and are obstacles to starting a healthy, worthwhile habit like running.

## Tricks for Dealing With Negative Thoughts During Runs

*"Even when you have gone as far as you can, and everything hurts, and you are staring at the specter of self-doubt, you can find a bit more strength deep inside you, if you look closely enough."*
-Hal Higdon, running coach

I wish I could say that every run produces a glorious runner's high, but we all know that it doesn't work that way. There will be plenty of times when you're running or racing and you'll start feeling discouraged and dismayed. So how do you turn it around and get yourself feeling confident and motivated to keep up your running habit? Here's what to do.

**Use a mantra.** Whether they're positive or negative, words can be very powerful during a run. If negative thoughts, such as "I feel tired" or "I'm not going to finish this race," keep intruding, they'll become a self-fulfilling prophecy. Repeat positive phrases such as, "I feel good" or "I'm feeling better" and pretty soon you'll start believing it.

**Run outdoors.** If you've ever thought that running outside makes you feel better mentally than running indoors, you're not imagining things. Research shows that even small doses of outdoor exercise can have a significant effect on mental health. In a meta-analysis of 10 studies, researchers at the University of Essex found that moving outdoors for even just five minutes improved mood and self-esteem.

**Run with positive people.** If someone in your running group complains frequently during runs, it can be very contagious and may turn your runs into a negative experience. You're probably even better off running alone (or with your dog!) than with someone who's going to bring you down. A good running friend will build you up, support you and remind you about all there is to love about running.

Seek out positive running partners — you'll be amazed at how quickly your runs fly by and how much more you enjoy them. And don't feel guilty about dropping the negative running partners. Listening to someone's incessant complaining is not a productive use of your time and energy.

**Be grateful.** When I'm feeling negative during a run, I think back to times when I was injured, and how frustrated and disappointed I was back then. I think about those who are not able to run and realize how lucky I am to be healthy enough to continue running. Or, I think about how going for a run is way better than plenty of other things, like going to the dentist or being stuck in traffic. Before I know it, I'm feeling more positive and grateful, and my run starts flying by.

**Smile and be friendly.** Smiling activates your endorphins, and it's really tough to feel stressed when you're smiling. If you feel strange just smiling at nothing, save your happy face for when you see someone along your route. Being a friendly runner or encountering one can usually snap me out of any foul mood I may be in. You'll be amazed at how some people react to a big smile or a simple hello from a passing runner. And the positive vibes you generate will help keep you motivated for the rest of your run.

**Think about your great runs.** If you're having a bad run, think back to one of those perfect runs you've had in the past when running felt so easy and effortless. Think about that run you did when the scenery was so beautiful, and you couldn't believe what was right in front of you. Remind yourself that there will be plenty more rewarding runs in the future.

# Chapter 15
# Bust Your Running Excuses

Sometimes you may have the best intentions to run, but something gets in the way. Often it's a busy schedules or bad weather to blame; while other times it's just lack of motivation. Being ready for these excuses and having specific strategies to battle each one can help you push past them and stick to your running habit.

### Fight the "I'm Too Busy" Excuse

*"Even if we are busy, we have time for what matters. And when we focus on what matters, we can build the lives we want in the time we've got."*
–Laura Vanderkam, time management expert

When I first became a mom, I had a tough time balancing my new parenting responsibilities with work obligations and personal time. Going for a run seemed to be the first thing to get cut from my list of priorities. After all, I was now responsible for another human being (gulp!) and I felt kind of selfish for wanting to run. Over time, I realized that not running as frequently as I had in the past meant that other areas of my life were suffering. I was more stressed-out, cranky and not as productive at work. I missed having that "me time," which was even more critical now that another human being was dependent on me. For my and my family's well-being and happiness, I realized that I HAD to find the time to run on a more regular basis. (Sidenote: My jogging stroller became a lifesaver during that period of my early motherhood years!)

I know I'm not alone in my struggles to find time to run. Lack of time is one of the most common reasons why people give up on running or just aren't able to run as much as they'd like. But it's possible to make some small tweaks to carve out more time to run.

For me, scheduling my weekly runs and running on Mondays, as discussed in the previous section, have been essential strategies for finding more time to run. Below are some other tips that I and other runners have used to make running a priority. Although some of these strategies may not work for everyone, I'm sure you'll find a few that can help you claim some more running time during your week. As running becomes more of a regular habit, you'll find that you're no longer saying, "I just don't have time to run."

**Take a good look at your schedule.** Look for wasted time during your week and find things that you can easily cut out of your schedule. For example, are you spending time at night on social media or watching TV? Use that time to run, or get to bed earlier so you can run in the morning.

**Run right after work.** Bring your running clothes to work and instead of hopping in the car or on a train at the end of the day, go for a run first. It'll be a great way to de-stress after a long day and you'll get the added bonus of missing the bulk of rush hour traffic.

**Get some help.** If you have kids, work it out with your significant other so that you can have coverage to fit your run in. Or do a kid swap with another parent so you can both get in some running time. Many gyms offer babysitting, so you can get in a treadmill run while someone is watching your children.

**Find 10 minutes.** A running habit can start small. Everyone can find 10 minutes to go for a short run or walk. Eventually you can add onto that mini habit and 10 minutes can turn into 30 minutes.

**Delegate**. Accept the fact that you can't do it all and look for ways you can farm out other tasks. Reassess the ways things are done at home and work. Can your spouse cook dinner sometimes? Can the kids help out with the laundry? Can you order things online that you're spending time shopping for? Are you doing things that don't actually need to get done?

**Learn to say, "No."** Take a look at your commitments and decide which ones are unnecessary or unimportant.

**Set running dates.** Plan to run with a friend or running group on a regular basis. Knowing that others are counting on you to be there will help you keep that commitment to run. And you'll be multi-tasking, since you also get to socialize during your run. The interaction will serve as a reward for running. If you have co-workers who run, see who's interested in a lunchtime or after-work run. You may find you can even have a "running meeting" with a colleague.

**Run while you wait.** Rather than cramming in an errand while your kid is at soccer practice or his piano lesson, go for a run. I always have extra running clothes and shoes in my trunk so I can sneak in a run if I have unexpectedly some extra time while shuttling my kids around to their activities.

## Have a Bad Weather Plan

*"If you haven't been exercising, your body will undoubtedly protest this change in its comfortable downhill direction. You won't like it at first. You may even hate it. But be proactive. Do it anyway. Even if it's raining on the morning you're scheduled to jog, do it anyway. 'Oh good! It's raining! I get to develop my willpower as well as my body!'"*
-Stephen Covey, author of *The Seven Habits of Highly Effective People*

Don't let excessive heat, rain or snow be an excuse for you to not run. It's possible to run in most weather conditions, as long as you take the proper precautions. Running in the rain is much more comfortable if you wear a hat with a brim to keep the rain off your face. Cold weather running can be invigorating and enjoyable, provided you're dressed for the weather. Visit your local running shop to get cold weather running shirts and pants, winter running socks, as well as a warm running hat and gloves.

Of course, sometimes it's just not safe or you may just not have the mental fortitude that day to run in some extreme weather conditions. That's OK – all runners have days like that. But you need to make sure you're prepared with a back-up plan so you don't blow off too many runs when bad weather hits.

I always prefer to run outside whenever possible, but I still belong to a gym so I have the option to run on a treadmill when it's icy, snowy, dangerously hot or too late/dark to run outside. I also have an outdated, squeaky treadmill at home that I refuse to get rid of because I still use it when we get so much snow that I can't drive to the gym. So I have a back-up plan for my back-up plan.

You don't need access to a treadmill to keep your running habit alive when the weather just isn't cooperating. You can do a home-based workout with some cardio such as jumping rope and stair-climbing, as well as some strengthening exercises. Even if you just work out for 20 minutes, you'll feel better that you didn't skip a day and it will help maintain the momentum of your running habit. And you can get right back to your regular running routine when the weather clears up.

## How to Beat the Running Blahs

*"There is an expression among even the most advanced runners that getting your shoes on is the hardest part of any workout."*
–Kathrine Switzer, women's running pioneer

Even if you have perfect conditions, sometimes getting those running shoes on can be tough. Here are some running motivation tricks to give yourself the push you need:

**Pick a race.** Having a deadline on the calendar gives many runners incentive to get out there. Following a training schedule for your race will also give structure to your running and renew your motivation every time you check off a workout.

**Do the five-minute test.** This is an old trick that I heard from another running coach. If you're having a hard time getting motivated and really feel yourself struggling when you start, tell yourself to run for another five minutes. If you're still feeling bad at that point, end your run and give yourself a rest day. You'll find that most of the time it was just a mental hurdle you needed to get over, and you'll continue running since you're already out there.

**Use motivating music.** Listening to some of your favorite songs can really help you get motivated to get running and keep moving once you get out there.

**Vary your running routes.** If you always run the same routes week after week, you may be bored, which can make it tough to get motivated. Switch things up and plan some new routes into different areas. Try some trail running, if you've never done that before. I love being able to step out my door and run, but sometimes it's totally worth it to drive to another location. A change of scenery and location will give you something to look forward to during your runs and add a new element to your training.

**Add variety to your workouts.** Boredom also happens if you're always doing the same distances, at the same paces. Mix it up with some interval workouts or some hill running. Throw some strengthening exercises into the middle of a run to change it up. When I'm running in a park, I'll sometimes stop at a bench or picnic table to do some step-ups, tricep dips, and push-ups for a couple minutes and then continue my run.

**Watch an inspiring movie.** Whether it's a movie about running, like *McFarlund, USA*, or something else motivational, watching an inspiring movie (before a run or during a treadmill run) can give you a big push to keep training.

**Think about your post-run self.** When you just don't feel like running, think about how you'll feel after you finish. Tell yourself that you'll feel healthier, stronger, and more focused. It's really hard to feel worse after a run. I can't think of a time when I actually regretted going for a run. But I can remember plenty of times when I was kicking myself for not going when I had the chance. If you're having a hard time motivating yourself to get out of bed, get off the couch or get out of that desk chair, think about your post-run self and get yourself to that feeling.

## **Beat Boredom**

*"The advice I have for beginners is the same philosophy that I have for runners of all levels of experience and ability – consistency, a sane approach, moderation and making your running an enjoyable, rather than dreaded, part of your life."*
-Bill Rodgers, four-time winner of Boston Marathon

Even the biggest running aficionados deal with bouts of boredom from time to time. Sometimes we need to revisit our running rituals and shake things up so they remain fresh. It's important to have several different boredom-busting strategies, since one isn't guaranteed to work all the time. And while listening to music and watching your favorite show are always great strategies for adding some excitement to a run, these ideas go beyond creating new playlists or binge-watching. Try some of these strategies the next time you're feeling bored while running:

**Brainstorm ideas.** Running can really help get the creative juices flowing. In the relaxed state of running, it's easy to clear your mind and really focus on a subject. I like to use my running time to think about ideas and plan. I think about upcoming vacations, new articles to write, meals to cook, emails I need to compose, activities for my kids to do or gift ideas for relatives or friends.

**Get distracted.** Try really paying attention to all the sights and sounds you're passing. This is usually pretty easy to do if you're running in a race and there are other runners, spectators and distractions around. When running in nature, paying attention to your surroundings can prevent boredom and also make you appreciate being able to run while surrounded by natural beauty. Personally, running near a body of water is almost always a peaceful experience for me.

**Run off some steam.** If I'm stressed or angry about something, running almost always makes me feel better. A running break helps me get away from the situation and think more clearly about it. And often the run gives me the perspective to realize it's not really something that I want to spend my time being angry or worried about. That angry email I was about to write before my run? It suddenly seems like not such a good idea after I've been able to chill out and gain perspective during my run.

**Focus on the workout and your performance.** Whenever I do a very structured workout, such as an interval workout or hill repeats, the time goes by very quickly. I don't get bored because I'm always changing and focusing on something different — the time, my pace, the recovery. If you typically do most of your runs at the same, easy pace or on flat courses, try mixing it up with some speed work or hills.

**Solve problems.** Running gives me uninterrupted, peaceful time to think deeply and productively about something I want to fix. With limited distractions, I'm able to really focus on the problem and brainstorm possible solutions.

**Alternate with another cardio machine.** If you're really bored on the treadmill, try breaking up your treadmill run by alternating with the bike or elliptical trainer. If you want to do a 40-minute cardio workout, run on the treadmill for 10 minutes and then jump on another machine for 10 minutes, and keep alternating until you've reached your total goal time.

If you have a treadmill at home and no other cardio machines, try running up and down the stairs or do jumping jacks for five minutes, in between running segments.

## How to Deal With Slowing Down as You Get Older

*"You don't stop running because you get old, you get old because you stop running."*
-Christopher McDougall, author of Born to Run

I often tell people, "You're never too told to start running," and I tell them about my mother, who ran her first marathon at age 62. Running is a safe, healthy exercise for people of any age. Personally, I hope to one day be that 80-year-old woman still running in races and having a blast.

Of course, slowing down is inevitable as runners age. As we get older, we lose muscle strength and aerobic capacity and we need more recovery time, so we just can't train and race at the same level. But don't let frustration with slower runs or race times be an excuse to break your running habit.

It helps to think about all the reasons why you fell in love with running in the first place. Maybe you really like the camaraderie and social aspects of running. Or, perhaps you love the health benefits and how you feel during and after a run.

If you feel like you need new motivation to keep running, try to mix things up to get more enjoyment out of running. Run with a group, do a relay race, sign up for a mud run or other theme race, try a new race distance, or run a race with a friend who's never done one before. You may be surprised at how much fun running can be when you're not so focused on your training and racing times.

## Focus on New Goals, Not Performance-Related

You can also try to set some goals for yourself that are not performance-related, such as staying injury-free, running a race for a charity, or doing a running streak for a certain amount of time. Taking the focus away from race times will help you enjoy running more and not be so bummed out about slowing down. You may find that you can still experience a lot of joy and sense of accomplishment from running beyond your race times.

Of course, if you're the type of runner who's very motivated by time goals, you can still set goals, but you need to make sure they're realistic. You need to redefine your definition of success and stop comparing yourself to your previous times, or other runners. In most cases, that's an unrealistic goal and you're just setting yourself up for disappointment. Instead of trying to beat your race personal record, aim to finish in the top half (or other percentage) of your age group. As you get older, you can still push yourself to achieve realistic time goals and feel satisfaction in achieving them.

## How to Be a More Resilient Runner

*"Running is a big question mark that's there each and every day. It asks you, 'Are you going to be a wimp or are you going to be strong today?'"*
-Peter Maher, Olympic marathon runner

We've all had those days when the answer to that question is, "I'm a wimp today." It's tempting to give into feelings of laziness and fear, but there are things you can do to make yourself more resistant to those urges and keep your running habit going strong. Here are a few ideas on how to be a more resilient runner:

**1. Focus on your weaknesses.** It sounds counterintuitive, but paying attention to your weak spots can help you get tougher. If you always fade on the hills, work on hill repeats. If your form falls apart when you get tired, do more core strengthening to avoid hunching over during the later miles. If you always struggle during the last few miles of a half or full marathon, work on it by picking up the pace at the end of your long runs.

Not only will you become stronger physically, but facing your weaknesses will improve your mental strength and confidence.

**2. Run with a purpose.** If you're running for the wrong reasons (like trying to impress someone) or for no reason at all, you're more likely to give up when things get tough. Figure out your personal running motivation, such as improving your health, setting new personal records, reaching new distances, or getting some peaceful alone time. Pick some specific running goals that relate to your motivation. Having that inner motivation means you'll care about what you're fighting for and you'll be more likely to tough it out.

**3. Confront your fears.** Are you scared to run in the rain? Do you worry about running in a crowded race? The best way to overcome your fears is to tackle them head-on. If you're really nervous about taking on a new running challenge, ask a friend to do it with you. I had wanted to do an obstacle course for a long time but only had the motivation and nerve when my sister-in-law asked me to do one with her. Had I given into my fears, I would have missed out on a very fun and inspiring experience.

Ask other runners how they deal with running anxiety and manage those situations. You may discover there was no reason to be worried and come out stronger on the other side.

# Chapter 16

# Prevent and Recover from Running Injuries

*"There is more to failing than picking yourself up out of the dust, brushing off the grime and trudging onward. For every defeat, there is a victory inside waiting to be let out if the runner can get past feeling sorry for himself."*
-Ron Daws, *The Self-Made Olympian*

Nothing can squash a running habit quite like an injury does. And many runners find that injuries hit at the worst possible time – right when they've gotten into a serious running groove and are feeling really good about their progress. Even though you may have the motivation and commitment to keep your habit going, your body just isn't cooperating.

Some runners assume that injuries are inevitable, but I know plenty of runners who have been running injury-free for years. The best approach to preventing running injuries is to be proactive and avoid behaviors that often lead to injury. Follow these injury prevention rules and you'll increase your odds of running injury-free.

**1. Wear the right shoes.** Finding the right pair of running shoes is one of the most important (and easiest!) steps you can take to prevent running injuries. Wearing the wrong shoes for your feet and running style can aggravate existing problems, causing pain in your feet, legs, knees or hips. Even just making sure you're wearing the correct size (should be at least 1/2 size bigger than your street shoe size) can prevent issues such as black toenails and blisters. Go to a specialty running shop where you can be properly fitted for running shoes, and replace them every 400 to 500 miles.

**2. Vary your running surfaces.** To give your joints and legs a break, do some of your runs on grass, dirt trails, and synthetic or dirt running tracks. Constantly running on concrete can lead to shin splints and other overuse injuries. Also, make sure you're running on a level surface. Running on a cambered (slanted) road can lead to overpronation (when your foot rolls inward) on one foot, which can eventually cause an injury.

Although the treadmill may not be your favorite surface for running, it's perfect for balanced and more cushioned running. It's a great option especially for new runners, those who are coming back from an injury or runners who are doing very high weekly mileage.

**3. Don't skip your warm-up or cooldown.** Getting your muscles warmed-up before you start a workout will help them stretch out and get longer. And muscles work more efficiently when they're longer, since they exert more force with less effort. Warmed-up muscles will also therefore be less prone to injury. Likewise, an easy cooldown can also help reduce injury risk. It gently brings back muscles to a resting state and will help speed recovery by helping to dissipate lactic acid after a hard run or race.

To warm-up before a run or race, do about 5 to 10 minutes of light aerobic exercise to loosen and warm up your muscles. Try walking briskly, marching, jogging slowly, or cycling on a stationary bike. You can also do some warm-up exercises such as jumping jacks, butt kicks or high knees. Make sure you don't rush your warm-up. After you finish your run, cool down by walking or slowly jogging for 5 to 10 minutes.

**4. Stretch after your runs.** Lack of flexibility can be a contributing factor in numerous overuse injuries, from Achilles tendinitis to shin splints. Tight muscles can't go through their range of motion properly, which may lead to improper form, discomfort and injuries.

The best time to stretch is after your runs, when your muscles are already warmed-up and elongated. Make stretching part of your post-run routine to help improve your flexibility and performance. You should especially focus on stretching your calves, hamstrings, quadriceps, hips and glutes, but don't forget about your upper body.

**5. Strength-train.** Regular strength-training helps to keep your body properly aligned and more injury-resistant. Strong core and hip muscles are the key to preventing many common running injuries, including knee injuries. You don't need to do intense strengthening workouts and build huge muscle mass to prevent injuries. Doing core, hip and lower-leg strength training two to three times a week will help you develop muscle balance, stability and proper alignment of your hips and legs.

**6. Ramp up slowly.** One of the most common causes of running injuries is doing too much, too soon, too quickly. Increase your mileage by no more than 10% each week. Beginners and those who've been injury-prone in the past should run every other day. You can use those off days in between to recover or cross train. Doing activities other than running, such as cycling, swimming, or yoga, allows you to build your fitness and strength, while giving your running muscles and joints a break.

**7. Listen to your body.** Most running injuries develop over time and send some warning signals, such as aches, consistent pain and soreness. It's up to you to pay attention to these warning signs and take action. If you feel pain that doesn't go away after you warm-up or you find yourself limping, don't push through your run – you'll only make your injury worse, or cause another injury due to overcompensation. Try RICE (Rest, Ice, Compression, Elevation) self-treatment and visit a doctor if you don't see much improvement after about a week off from running.

**8. Use injury prevention tools.** There's a lot you can do to keep minor aches or pains from turning into a full-blown running injury. Icing a sore spot with an ice pack or a bag of frozen peas for 10 to 15 minutes after a long run can make a big difference. If you're feeling pain on the bottom of your foot, freeze a water bottle and roll your foot on top of it. You can use massage tools such as a foam roller, the Stick or even a tennis ball to roll out any areas that feel tight post-run.

## Recharge With Rest Days

Even the most experienced runners need some down time. The American College for Sports Medicine recommends one to two rest days per week to reduce injury risk. Resting also gives your body a chance to recover, repair itself and readapt to the training load. You'll find that you'll actually feel better and stronger during your runs.

Rest days also give you a mental break, reducing your chances of feeling burned out and bored of running. We all have limited amounts of mental and physical energy and if we keep drawing on our reservoir of energy without any replenishment (rest), we'll eventually burn out and break down.

I strongly encourage you to take at least one day off from exercise every week. When you do it is up to you. Some runners like to rest on Fridays, since they may be tired by the end of the week and want to gear up for a longer weekend run. Try to plan your rest days in the beginning of the week, just like you do your weekly runs, so you'll know when that recharging day is coming.

One day of complete rest is sufficient for most runners, but that doesn't mean that you need to run on the other days. I highly recommend doing some form of activity on the other days to keep your habit formation moving forward.

Biking, swimming, spinning, walking, yoga or strength-training are all good cross-training options that will help deepen the groove of your exercise habit. I like to do a boot camp class or yoga on my non-running days, but you should choose an activity that you enjoy so you'll look forward to it. I often run by myself, so I like doing group exercise classes on my non-running days to mix things up.

## 5 Warning Signs of Running Injuries

Runners often feel pain come and go, sometimes very quickly. I tend to panic when I feel a soreness in my shin or other area, and start thinking about the worst case scenario. Most often, the pain goes away just as quickly as it started. But what about the pains that don't go away or get worse during runs? How do you know when you're on the brink of a running injury? Here are some ways to determine whether your pain is just a little ache or a warning sign of an injury. Listening to your body and paying attention to these signs can help you prevent a minor issue from turning into a full-blown injury.

**1. The pain gets worse as you keep running.** We've all had those runs where something feels a little tight or uncomfortable when you start your run, but then it goes away after we're warmed-up. If your pain feels the same or gets progressively worse as you continue running, stop running and take a few days off to see if you notice any improvement.

**2. You're changing your stride.** A minor ache or pain shouldn't force you to change your gait when you're running. If you've done your 5 to 10-minute warm-up before your run and your stride is still off, take a couple of days off from running and see if that makes a difference.

**3. It's affecting your performance.** If you're slow or sluggish and can't figure out why, give yourself some additional rest and recovery time. You won't lose fitness over a couple of days of rest.

**4. The area is sore and swollen.** If you've recently done a long run or an intense workout, some muscle soreness after running is normal. But if there's also swelling where you're feeling pain, the inflammation may be a sign that something's not right. Ice it (15 to 20 minutes every 3 to 4 hours) and rest for a couple of days.

**5. You're feeling pain even when you're not running.** Is the pain causing you to limp when you're just walking around or sitting for a long period of time? If that's the case and you find that the pain is affecting your daily activities, you should get it checked out by a health care professional.

## Should I Ice or Heat My Running Injury?

Applying ice or heat can provide relief for many injuries. Depending on your injury, though, you should use these treatments at different times. Basically, you shouldn't keep going back and forth between a bag of ice and a heating pad, which I know a lot of runners are guilty of doing!

Here's a guide to when to use hot or cold therapy on post-run pain:

## When to Use Cold Therapy

When you're first injured, ice is a better choice than heat. It can reduce both pain and inflammation of an injury and is usually helpful for the first 24 to 48 hours after an injury. You can use ice immediately after sustaining an acute injury, such as a sprained ligament or strained muscle. You can also use ice if you've re-aggravated a chronic injury, such as plantar fasciitis or shin splints. Cold baths or swimming/sitting in cold water can also help with muscle recovery after running a marathon or completing a long training run.

**What to Use:** You can use an ice pack, a plastic bag filled with ice; a bag of frozen vegetables; or even a frozen water bottle, which is especially good for pain on the bottom of the foot. Make sure that you place a towel between the ice and your skin – don't apply it directly. Although ice therapy is generally safe and effective, don't use ice for longer than 20 minutes at a time because of the risk of damage to your nerves and skin.

**How Long:** Ice for 15 to 20 minutes for three to five times a day, if possible. For acute injuries, ice the first 24 to 48 hours after the injury. For chronic injuries, ice when you've re-aggravated the injury and are feeling pain.

## When to Use Heat Therapy

Following the first 24 to 48 hours of an injury, heat can increase blood flow to the injury, which may help promote healing. Heat also serves as a muscle relaxer, which can help with pain relief. If you have a tender or tight spot that's been bothering you for a little while, applying heat before you run or workout can help loosen your muscle and relax the area.

**What to Use:** Use a heating pad or a towel soaked with hot water. Place the pad on or wrap the towel around the affected area.

**How Long:** Before you head out for a run, apply heat for 5 to 10 minutes. If you have a tight area after a long period of sitting or staying in the same position, you can also apply heat for 10 to 15 minutes for some relief.

## How to Come Back from a Running Injury

Coming back from an injury can be a frustrating, slow process, but it's critical that you don't try to rush it. That can be extremely difficult, especially if you've gotten into a good running groove or you're training for a big race. You may assume that taking time off will put your race in jeopardy but, in reality, pushing through an injury can make it worse and keep you sidelined for a lot longer than if you took the right steps at the injury onset. So it's important to be patient, embrace your time off from running and understand that rest is an important part of your recovery process.

**If you've been out less than a week:**

You should be able to get right back to your training without losing any ground. Take it easy for your first couple of runs back. If you feel good during those runs, it's safe to return to your normal training schedule. You may feel a bit sluggish at first, but it should only take one or two runs before you're feeling like your old self.

One important caveat: Don't try to make up the miles that you missed. If you try to cram all your missed workouts into a short period of time, you could be at risk for re-injuring yourself or causing another overuse injury and you'll end up sidelined yet again.

**If you've been out one to two weeks:**

You're going to lose at least some fitness, even if you've been cross-training on a regular basis.

Go easy when you first return to running because if you run too hard, you risk re-injuring yourself. Start at about half the distance you were running before your injury. You should be able to build back to your previous level in two to four weeks.

**If you've been out more than two weeks:**
You need to be more conservative when you get back to running. Even if you were running with no walk breaks before your injury, you might need to start with a run/walk strategy, alternating between intervals of running and walking. Doing run/walk will allow you to build your fitness safely, without all the pounding of running. As you improve your endurance, you'll be able to extend your run intervals and reduce your walking time.

During your first couple of weeks back, take a day off after every running day. Running every day may lead to a re-injury or a new overuse injury. For your weekly mileage, you'll need to gradually work up to your previous level. And don't keep making jumps in your mileage. It's good to get comfortable with a specific weekly mileage by staying there for a couple weeks, and then bump up your distance.

If you're training for a specific race and trying to get back on schedule, supplement your running with another cardio exercise, such as biking or swimming.

## How to Deal With the Emotional Impact of a Running Injury

Aside from causing some physical pain, a running injury can also take a big emotional toll on runners. You may feel unhappy, frustrated and more anxious, since running was an outlet for your stress. But it doesn't have to be that way. Rather than feeling sorry for yourself, you can make the most of your recovery and put yourself in a good position to get back to your running habit when you've recovered. Follow these strategies:

**Try not to adopt a "woe-is-me" attitude.** A positive, optimistic outlook can help speed up your recovery. It helps to surround yourself with uplifting people. If someone has negative energy and doesn't understand why you're so bummed about your injury, now might be a good time to limit your exposure to that person. Talk to friends and relatives who can sympathize with your situation.

**Stay active.** Keeping active can also help you deal with the emotional struggles of a running injury. Talk to your doctor or physical therapist about recommendations for safe cross-training activities during your recovery. Some good choices are usually low-impact activities such as yoga, swimming, strength-training or deep water running. The physical activity will help prevent feelings of stress, sadness, and anger. And you'll feel better knowing that you're still burning lots of calories and maintaining some of your fitness.

**Keep up your routine.** Although you can't run, you should still try to stick to your running habit rituals as much as possible. If you're typically a morning runner, go for a walk or do strength-training in the morning. Keeping up your habit of going to the gym or being active outside will also help ease the transition back to your running routine. Try to do something every day that will keep your running habit formation going.

**Be patient.** Make sure you're being realistic in your goals and expectations and not rush the recovery process. I've seen many runners start running again when their injury isn't quite healed and they end up re-injuring themselves. Be smart and patient and you'll soon be back up and running. Keep telling yourself that your injury is only temporary and it will pass.

**See the positive.** The silver lining of any injury is that it does give you a better appreciation for running. You'll be much less likely to take running for granted. You'll strengthen your resolve to maintain your running habit. And you'll pay much more attention to injury prevention steps and warning signs that can help you avoid another injury in the future.

## Can I Run With a Cold?

Even something as minor as a common cold can thwart your running habit. One of the most common questions I hear from runners who I coach is, "Is it safe to run with a cold?" The answer, as is the case with many running-related questions is, "It depends."

Let your symptoms be your guide when determining if you can run with a cold. Use the above/below neck rule. If your symptoms are above your neck, such as runny or stuffy nose, sneezing, itchy eyes or sore throat, it's safe to run. You may want to slow down your usual pace and drink some more water during your run, but you should generally feel OK. If your symptoms are below your neck, such as chest congestion, upset stomach or diarrhea, then you should rest and wait until those symptoms pass before attempting to run.

## How Runners Can Avoid Getting Sick

Although it's possible to run through mild cold symptoms, it's much easier to avoid getting sick in the first place. Try these strategies to stay healthy, boost your immune system and avoid a cold being an annoying obstacle to your running habit:

**Wash your hands frequently.** Washing your hands with soap and warm running water is one of the best and easiest things you can do to stay healthy. Be especially vigilant when you're in a public place like a restaurant, your gym or any crowded area.

**Get plenty of sleep.** Sleep deprivation can make you more susceptible to colds and other illnesses. Getting proper sleep — at least seven to eight hours per night — will boost your immune system. Bonus: You'll also run better when you're well-rested.

**Maintain a balanced diet.** Get plenty of fruits and vegetables, which contain antioxidants, and limit your saturated fats.

**Drink water.** Staying hydrated is important for illness prevention, so make sure that you're drinking plenty of water during the day and hydrating during exercise. You'll know you're properly hydrated if your urine is light yellow.

**Don't skip the tapering period.** If you're running a long distance race, such as a marathon, it's important to cut back your mileage in the two to three weeks before your race. This tapering period will allow your immune system to recover from all the hard training you've been doing and make you less susceptible to a pre-race cold.

**Be diligent after your race, too.** Many long distance runners come down with a cold after an endurance event because their body's immune system is busy repairing the damage rather than fighting off infections. So cold prevention strategies are especially critical during the three to four days following your race.

# PART FOUR

# GIVE BACK (AND RECEIVE MORE)

*"Service to a just cause rewards the worker with more real happiness and satisfaction than any other venture of life."*
-Carrie Chapman Catt, American social reformer

## Chapter 17
## Ways Runners Can Do Good

*"From what we get, we can make a living. What we give, however, makes a life."*
-Arthur Ashe, tennis great

Do you know which activity can put you in a better mood, reduce your stress, and enrich your sense of purpose in life? I'm not talking about running although, on most days, I get those same benefits when I go for a run.

It's volunteering that can make us happier, motivated and less stressed-out, according to recent research. Donating your time and skills is not only helpful for the recipients, but you're likely to reap a lot of benefits as well.

Indeed, as a volunteer coach for my kids' track team, I truly believe that I've gotten so much more from my experience than I've ever given. Seeing the kids' faces light up and watching their confidence soar as they cross the finish line, nail a long jump or complete their longest distance ever is an instant mood-booster. It also helps reinforce my own running habit and reminds me of running's benefits and all the reasons why I love the sport.

Volunteering within the running community also helps you feel more connected to that network, which will give you a huge motivation boost. So it's a total win-win for everyone involved. If you're looking for ways to serve the running community or your community at large, here are some ideas for giving back.

**1. Volunteer at a race.** Race organizers really depend on volunteers to keep races running smoothly. They also help keep the price of race entry fees down, since it would cost a ton of money to pay all the people who work at races. As a volunteer, you can help with race registration, crowd control, passing out water or the very fun and desirable job of placing medals around finishers' necks. If you've never run a race before, volunteering is an excellent way to test the waters before you sign up for your first race.

To sign up to volunteer at a race, go to the race's website and look for the volunteer opportunities. Or, reach out to the race director. If you're interested in running the race AND volunteering, it's possible to do both by volunteering before or after the race. You may even get a free race entry!

**2. Clean up a local trail or park.** If there's a trail or park near you that could use some cleaning-up, grab some garbage bags and a pair of gloves and get to it. Ask your running friends if they want to join you. If you have kids, get them involved. Better yet, if your kids are in Girl Scouts or Boy Scouts, plan an organized clean-up effort with your kids' troop.

**3. Coach or mentor other runners.** You don't have to be a running expert to help coach or mentor other runners. If you have a friend or family member who has shown some interest in running, share your experience with them and help them get started the way you did. (More tips on how to mentor a new runner are included later in this chapter.) Look for volunteer opportunities to help coach runners, such as a youth running team. Girls on the Run, a national running program for girls in grades 3 to 8, is always looking for volunteer coaches.

**4. Run for a charity.** Whatever your favorite causes or charities may be, there's a way that you can run to support it. Some smaller races, such as 5Ks, are organized as fundraising events for a specific charity or cause. Part of your entry fee goes to the cause and you can also fundraise more by getting people to sponsor you.

Many big races, such as popular marathons, offer charity runner spots, which means you can fundraise a certain amount of money for a cause to get guaranteed entry into the race. If you're interested in a specific race, look at the charity section on the race's website to learn about their designated charities.

If your favorite charity doesn't organize a fundraiser race or have charity spots, you can still raise money on their behalf by using a fundraising website such as Crowdwise. Or use the CharityMiles app, which allows runners to earn up to 25¢ per mile for their charity.

**5. Donate your gently-used running clothes and gear.** If you have piles of gently-used running clothes just sitting in your closet, donate them to charities such as Goodwill or Salvation Army, or list them on Freecycle.org. Animal shelters could use old race T-shirts. Ask running friends if they'd like any of your old running gear that you no longer use. I know some running groups do running gear swaps among members so runners can give their old gear and gadgets a new life.

If you don't like to save your race medals, you can donate them to Medals4Mettle, a non-profit organization that facilitates the gifting of marathon, half marathon and triathlon finishers' medals to children and adults fighting debilitating diseases.

## Fundraising Tips for Charity Runners

As a coach for the Leukemia and Lymphoma Society's Team in Training for the past 15 years, I see first-hand how being part of a charity team can reinforce a running habit and boost runners' motivation and love of the sport.

Even if you don't want to join a charity team, you can fundraise on your own or with some friends or co-workers. Having a greater cause and purpose for your running will help keep you motivated and committed to your running habit.

Of course, fundraising can be a daunting, intimidating process. I've talked to a lot of runners who were way more nervous about raising the minimum amount than actually running the race. Here are some tips to help navigate the process and achieve fundraising success:

**1. Start early.** Get going with your fundraising as soon as you can. If you start early, you'll be able to reach your minimum sooner and not stress about it. An added bonus is that starting your fundraising will boost your motivation to train, since you'll feel more committed to your race. Each donation will feel like a reward for your training efforts, so it will help you establish your running habit loop.

**2. Create a fundraising website.** Many people prefer the convenience of making online donations, and most charities offer fundraisers the opportunity to set up a personalized website. Make sure you take the steps to set it up and personalize it. You don't have to be a computer expert to do it – it's usually a very easy, straight-forward process.

Share your personal connection to the cause, why donations are so critical and how the money is used. Include photos of any personal honorees and/or of yourself before, after or during a training run.

**3. Set your fundraising goal for higher than your minimum.** If you have a minimum fundraising amount that you need to reach in order to earn a race entry or receive another incentive, set your goal for higher than that amount. When potential donors see that you have a lot of money to raise, they're more likely to make a donation and give generously.

**4. Write a fundraising letter.** One of the quickest and easiest ways to raise money is to ask everyone you know to donate. Write a fundraising letter explaining what you're doing and email it to your contacts, everyone from friends and family members to co-workers and members of clubs you belong to. You'll be surprised at who donates. Some people you don't know very well may have a close connection to the cause that you're supporting and be very happy and grateful for the opportunity to support you.

**5. Customize your letter.** The charity you're supporting may give you same sample fundraising letters (and I've also included some examples later in this chapter), but don't use a template word-for-word. Make it your own by sharing your reasons for why you care about the particular charity and why you're doing the race. Include information about the charity (statistics, articles, and videos, for example) so your potential donors can find out how their money can make a difference. Don't forget to include how people can donate!

**6. Form a team.** Fundraising as a team can be more effective – and fun! Recruit co-workers or friends to join your team. You can support and encourage each other's running and fundraising efforts, and plan fundraising events together. Ask the organization you're supporting if there are incentives or programs for fundraising teams. For example, they may be able to set up a group fundraising page for your team so you can pool your donations. An added bonus of being part of a team is that you can all train together and keep each other on track with your training.

**7. Use social media.** Post your fundraising website link on Facebook, Twitter and other social media that you use to get your message out. Ask donors if it's OK to acknowledge their donation and thank them publicly on Facebook or other social media. Seeing you thank donors publicly may inspire or remind your other connections to make a contribution.

**8. Use email.** After you send out your initial email, send a follow-up one a few weeks later with an update on your progress. Send another reminder email to your list a couple weeks after that. Finally, send an update email after your race, thanking those who donated and encouraging those who haven't to make a donation. Put reminders on your calendar to send out the emails, so you don't forget. Add the URL for your fundraising website to your email signature, as a reminder to anyone you email that you're still raising money.

**9. Plan a fundraising event.** You don't need to plan a huge gala to raise money. A fundraising event could be as simple as hosting a dinner party or wine tasting event at your home and asking guests to donate. See if a local restaurant will offer a percentage of its sales for a certain night to your cause. Get friends and local businesses to donate items so you can do a raffle at your event. When you send out your invitations, don't forget to include your fundraising link, so those who can't attend can still donate to your cause.

**10. Hold a yard sale.** Do you have a lot of clutter in your closets and garage? Clear them out and sell any unwanted items at a yard sale. Ask friends and relatives if they have items they want to contribute to your sale. Some people may not have the means to make a financial contribution to your fundraising efforts but are happy to help in other ways. If you don't want to organize a yard sale, try selling your used stuff at local consignment shops, on craigslist or eBay, or through social media.

**11. Get donations matched.** Find out if your company will match all or part of the donations that you raise. When people donate, ask them if their company has a matching gift program. For many companies, the matching gift process is as simple and easy as filling out a form.

**12. Have a bake sale.** Sell some baked goods at work, at your yard sale or fundraising event. Or do it outside a local store, if they allow it. You can put out a collection jar for those who want to donate money, but don't what to buy any sweets. Get pamphlets from the organization and let donors know how their donation will make a difference. Make sure you also have your fundraising link handy for people who want to make a credit card donation.

**13. Keep asking.** Don't be shy or embarrassed to remind people to make a donation. Some of your friends and relatives may have every intention of contributing to your fundraising efforts, but completely forgot or just haven't gotten around to it yet. Send them an update about your fundraising and training progress (photos are also fun to share) and let them know that it's not too late to donate. They'll appreciate the reminder.

## Sample Fundraising Letters

Here are a few samples of fundraising letters. You can also check with the organization you're supporting for additional letters. The most effective fundraising letters are written from the heart. Share your personal reasons for running the race and choosing the charity you're fundraising for, as well as your other motivations for running the race. Mention the names of any personal honorees who you're running in honor or memory of, and offer to run for others.

Dear Friends and Family,

I'm doing more than just running in this year's Susan G. Komen Washington, D.C. Race for the Cure.

I'm fundraising because the Washington, D.C. Metro Area still has one of the highest breast cancer mortality rates in the nation. And I believe that where you live should not determine whether you live.

I'm also raising funds because [inset your personal connection to the cause]. If you also have a personal connection, I'd be thrilled and honored to add your honoree to my list of people I'm running in honor of!

I've set my personal goal at $[insert your goal amount] and I'm asking for your help to reach my goal. You can give online, safely and securely, at [insert your link]

Up to 75 percent of the Komen Washington, D.C. Race for the Cure's net income stays in the Washington, D.C. Metropolitan Area to fund breast cancer screening, treatment and education programs through the National Capital Region Grant Program. The remaining 25 percent will go to fund national research programs.

Thank you in advance for your support. Your generosity saves lives!

Sincerely,
[Insert Your Name]

P.S. Please ask your employer if they will double your donation through a matching gift program!

Dear Friends and Family,

As a participant with the Leukemia and Lymphoma Society's Team in Training, I've had the honor of meeting many people who have been affected by blood cancers. Some are survivors with incredible stories of beating cancer, some are currently fighting the disease, and others are relatives and friends who run and fundraise in honor or memory of their loved ones. Not a week goes by when I don't hear a story about someone who lost their battle, or has had a recurrence. Their stories are a reminder that we need to keep fighting and raising money to find a cure.

So much amazing progress has been made in the fight against cancer…but we still have a long way to go. Yes, childhood leukemia now has an almost 90% cure rate, but that means that 10% of parents who hear their child's diagnosis will one day lose him or her to the disease. Someday there will be a cure, but we're not there yet. Our work will be done when every cancer diagnosis has a happy ending!

This year I'm fundraising for and running the [insert race name] on [insert race date] in support and honor of all those currently fighting leukemia, lymphoma, and myeloma. Please join me in this fight and help me prevent other people from losing their loved ones to these terrible diseases! The money you donate will help the Leukemia and Lymphoma Society fund valuable research and provide essential patient services. Visit my website to make a 100% tax-deductible donation: [insert your link]

Any donation – no matter how small – can truly make a difference. When a cure is finally found, you will be able to say that you were part of it! Thanks in advance for your support!
In appreciation,
[Insert Your Name]

Dear [Insert Name],

This year, I'm participating in the Via Marathon. I'll run with hundreds of other men, women and children for Via of the Lehigh Valley, a non-profit organization that provides services for children and adults with disabilities. Via provides therapeutic services for children, employment solutions for adults and helps people live a life of significance in the community.

Everyone deserves the opportunity to succeed and through your support, Via provides opportunities and resources every day for children and adults with disabilities. Via is committed to a mission of success for the people they serve, but they can't do it without our help.

I have chosen to participate because [insert your personal reasons for running]. I've never run a marathon before, but this cause is so important to me and I'm up for the challenge!

My team of family members and friends have agreed to raise at least [insert your dollar goal]. So we need your help. Please make a donation today: [insert personal webpage].

The opportunity to succeed for each child and adult begins with you. Thanks in advance for your support! I truly appreciate your support and promise to keep you updated on my fundraising and training progress!

With love and gratitude,
[Insert Your Name]

## **Acts of Kindness for Runners**

Extending kindness to someone, whether it's a loved one or a total stranger, can be a heart-warming and satisfying experience for everyone involved. And, ideally, one act of kindness will lead to a chain reaction of kind gestures.

When your act of kindness is connected to running, not only will you feel satisfied about doing a good deed, you'll have lots of positive feelings about running as well. A nice gesture towards a fellow runner can make you feel more connected to the sport and the running community. Your act of kindness can be a reward that reinforces your running habit.

Here are some random acts of kindness that are specific to runners. Refer back to this list when you feel like your running habit and your heart can use a little pick-me-up.

1. Check in on a running friend who's training for a big race and see how her training is going.

2. Offer to give directions to that runner in the park who looks lost.

3. Pass out paper towels during a race. Many runners will be grateful to be able to wipe their sweat or blow their nose.

4. Respect fellow runners by following the rules of wherever you're running, such as staying to the correct side of a running path or keeping your dog on a leash if you're running with him.

5. Send a running friend a good luck text or email for their upcoming race.

6. Give out ice pops to runners during a very hot race. (Or hand warmers during a frigid one.) They'll be incredibly grateful!

7. Thank charity runners in a race for raising money and awareness for a good cause.

8. Cheer for random strangers at a race, not just those you know running it. Make funny spectator signs so runners will get a laugh as they pass you.

9. Reach out to a running buddy who's injured and upset that she can't run or had to defer a race.

10. Congratulate running friends when they post a status or a photo about their running progress on social media.

11. Get to know new people in your running group. It can be awkward and intimidating to join a group without knowing anyone. Make newbies feel comfortable by being friendly and welcoming.

12. Share your running snacks. If you're doing a long run with a group, offer some of your running nutrition to others.

13. Thank the volunteers at races. They've been on their feet for a long time, too!

14. Donate your gently-used running clothes and gear. Give them to a local charity or offer them to running friends who you know could use them.

15. Say thank you to a running coach or someone else who gave you running instruction or encouraged you to start running. Even if you haven't spoken to the person in a long time, they'll love hearing a thank you from a former athlete.

16. Congratulate the runners who cross the finish line near you. Let them know that they helped you push to the finish.

17. Offer high-fives to the kids cheering or passing out water during a race you're running.

18. Smile and say hello to other runners or fitness walkers when you pass them. Give them a compliment such as, "Looking good!"

19. Organize a running shoe collection drive at your gym, office or at a race. You can donate the shoes to an organization that collects used running shoes.

20. Get to know regulars you see on your running route. Ask the woman walking her dog every morning for her (and her dog's) name, so you can personally greet her when you see her. People love the sound of their own name.

21. Send a thank you email to the race director of a race that you enjoyed. He or she will truly appreciate the positive feedback.

22. Take photos of friends while they're running a race and share them, along with a congratulatory note, after the race.

## Help a New Runner, Help Yourself

*"Help others achieve their dreams and you will achieve yours."*
-Les Brown, motivational speaker

If you have someone in your life, whether it's a friend, family member or co-worker, who's looking for some running support and guidance, you should definitely consider lending a hand. You'll both benefit. Your trainee will reap the healthy benefits of exercise, from stress relief to weight loss. And your motivation to run will improve as you reaffirm your enthusiasm and inspiration for running.

You may also be inspired to learn more about running, as those who mentor runners or other athletes find that they understand the principles of training better as they explain them to others. It's OK if you're still fairly new to running! You can still be a supportive and helpful influence. Here are ways to offer a new runner some help.

**1. Start slow.** Get them started with a little bit of running or run/walking, and gradually increase the distance. Have them follow a basic training schedule that's appropriate for their level. If they do too much too soon, they may get sore (or injured), get discouraged and want to throw in the towel.

Don't push your newbie runner through pain or discomfort, especially during the first few weeks. Make sure they know to stay at a comfortable, conversational pace. They shouldn't be huffing or puffing.

**2. Share your mistakes.** We were all new runners at some point, and it'll be helpful for your friend to hear about mistakes and setbacks you had when you were starting out. She'll be more likely to stick with her running if she knows it's normal to make mistakes or feel discouraged sometimes.

**3. Go shopping together.** New runners may be confused and feel a little overwhelmed picking out the right running shoes or gear. Take them to your favorite running gear shops, encourage them to get a running gait analysis and help them navigate the shoe, clothing and gear choices. Tell him or her about your favorite water bottles, watches, socks and running clothes.

**4. Pick a race.** Having a race, like a 5K, will keep BOTH of you motivated. Even if you don't want to run the race together, you can hang out before the race and after you finish. And then plan a way to celebrate together, like going for breakfast after the race, so you have a reward to look forward to. Make sure you take some photos together before and after the race, so you can look back and be reminded of the fun and achievements.

**5. Run together.** Of course you don't have to buddy up for every run, but try to get together to run occasionally. If your friend is much slower than you, stick to his or her pace. Or, if you belong to the same gym, run on side-by-side treadmills so pace isn't an issue! If it's not feasible to run together, see if you can help him or her find a local running group or training program in her area so that she has others to run with. Text or talk after your runs so you can keep each other up-to-date on your progress.

# Chapter 18
# Be Grateful

*"Running has always been a relief and a sanctuary — something that makes me feel good, both physically and mentally. For me it's not so much about the health benefits. Those are great, but I believe that the best thing about running is the joy it brings to life."*
-Kara Goucher, U.S. Olympic distance runner

You may have already heard about the numerous benefits of gratitude. Thousands of studies have shown that practicing gratitude can help you feel more content and less stressed, more optimistic and less anxious. Being grateful about running can also be a powerful, motivating force that keeps pushing your running habit forward.

When I'm running, I often think about the reasons I'm grateful for running. I love the peace and calmness that running brings me when I'm feeling stressed. Running allows me to hit the pause button on everything else that's going on in my life. From the moment I tie my running shoes, I'm no longer a mother, a wife, a coach, a writer – I'm just a runner. I can focus on the sound of my feet hitting the pavement and let my mind wander to wherever it wants to go. When I return from a run, I feel refreshed, re-energized and more confident to tackle my to-do list and face whatever problems emerge.

I'm grateful that running allows me to experience nature in all its beauty. When I'm running on the roads or on trails, I pay more attention to the sights, sounds and smells of nature. I have the time and patience to listen to the leaves crunching under my feet and spot the crocuses popping up through the soil.

I'm grateful for running and the bonds that it's helped me form and strengthen with family members and friends, old and new. Brad and I are both runners and, although we don't frequently run together, running gives us some common ground. We support each other through the highs and lows of running. The shared experiences – from crazy road trips to epic long runs – that I've had with my running friends have created memories and bonds to last a lifetime.

My mom started running several years ago and our relationship has deepened as we've run races together, swapped running tips, cheered for each other at races, and laughed about embarrassing running mishaps. Some of my fondest running memories, from both childhood and adult life, are seeing her face and hearing her cheer as I approached a finish line.

I'm grateful that running keeps me healthy and reminds me not to take my health for granted. I love being a healthy role model for my kids and showing them that exercise is fun AND good for you.

**TO DO: Figure out why you're grateful for running.**

Although not all runners' reasons to be grateful are the same, we can all find things about running that make us thankful for the ability to get out there and move. Find your reasons to be grateful and remind yourself of them when your motivation has hit rock bottom. Write them down in your training journal or a gratitude journal if that makes you remember them more. Make sure you're being intentional and specific when practicing gratitude; otherwise, it's not as effective.

## Chapter 19
## Love Running — For Good

*"Running should be a lifelong activity. Approach it patiently and intelligently, and it will reward you for a long, long time."*
-Michael Sargent, runner

Like any long-term relationship, my relationship with running has its ups and downs – and I'm not talking about hill repeats. Although I usually look forward to my runs, there are times when I'm really busy and running feels like another chore on an endless to-do list. Running starts to irritate me a little. I feel like I'm doing a lot of work with not much in return. The passion slightly fades, my eyes start to wander, and I'm envious of non-runners' freedom to not have to worry about scheduling long runs when they're having a really rough week or are going on vacation.

As anyone who's ever been in a committed relationship can attest, relationships are more successful when you focus on being a nurturing partner and paying attention to your significant other. The same can be said for running – the more committed I am to running, the more I'll be rewarded for my devotion and the less likely I am to take running for granted.

Whenever I start to question my relationship with running, I remind myself of the reasons why I fell in love with running in the first place and how my life is better because of running. I talk to running friends about what keeps them going. I'll pick up a book such as Haruki Murakami's *What I Talk About When I Talk About Running* or Donald Buraglio's *The Running Life*, which are both great perspectives on why people run and how it can be life-changing.

I think about not only running's physical and mental benefits, but of all the people I've met through running and memories made along the way. I remember times that I couldn't run because of injury, or I'll think about others who can't run because of physical limitations. That changes my focus from resentment to appreciation and gets me motivated to get back on the road.

# Conclusion

*"Move out of your comfort zone. You can only grow if you are willing to feel awkward and uncomfortable when you try something new."*
-Brian Tracy

## Dos and Don'ts for Running Habit Formation

It's normal to feel a bit overwhelmed or uncomfortable if you're brand-new to running. Try to take it one day at a time, one step at a time. Here's a quick refresher of some of the major tips and tricks for starting and maintaining your running habit.

### Here's what to DO:

• Get fitted for the right running shoes. You'll feel more comfortable and reduce your injury risk.

• Figure out your running cues, or triggers, that will signal you to go for a run.

• Determine some appropriate rewards for your runs, so you can create the habit loop of cue --> run --> reward and get your running habit into a deep groove.

• Follow a training schedule. Knowing exactly what you're supposed to do each day will keep you moving forward.

• Tell people about your running habit. You'll feel much more accountable and committed to your running.

- Start with a mini habit. Even five minutes of running a day can help you establish a solid running habit.

- Plan your runs for the week on Sunday. Schedule your runs on your calendar, set reminders for yourself and plan running dates. Make running part of your regular schedule so it's much harder to blow off.

- Run on Mondays. Get the week started on the right foot with a run.

- Track your progress and make it visible. Record your workouts in a training journal, on a calendar, in an app or whatever works for you.

- Run in the morning when you can. Morning runners are more consistent than evening runners.

- Find a running group. Group motivation is huge.

- Be prepared for setbacks and obstacles. They will happen. If you're expecting them, they're easier to manage and overcome.

- Create a positive environment. Hang with positive people, read uplifting books, watch inspiring movies and post positive quotes. Keep your self-talk positive.

- Give back to the sport of running – you'll undoubtedly get back way more than you give and be motivated to keep going.

- Remind yourself of all the reasons you started running and why you're grateful to be able to run.

- Visit **run-for-good.com** for even more inspiration and practical running advice to keep your running habit going.

## Here's what NOT to:

• Don't think ALL or nothing. Even a 10-minute run will deepen the groove of your running habit and keep you moving forward.

• Don't neglect other healthy habits. Get plenty of rest, eat healthy and reduce stress.

• Don't get too ambitious and sign up for a marathon as a brand-new runner. Think baby steps.

• Don't give up because you had a temporary setback such as illness, injury or lack of motivation or energy.

• Don't give into the "I'm too busy" excuse. Remember: We make time for the things that matter.

• Don't run or spend a lot of time with negative people. Don't listen to people who tell you that you'll get injured. Seek out positive friends who support you and your goals.

# Training Schedules

## 5K Beginner Training Schedule

This six-week 5K training program is designed for beginner run/walkers who want to build up to running a 5K (3.1 miles). This training schedule is a run/walk to continuous running program. Each week, you'll make small increases in your running distance while making slight decreases in your walking intervals. At the end of six weeks, you'll be ready to run the 5k distance without any walking breaks. (Although if you want to take walking breaks during the race, that's fine, too!)

To start this training schedule, you should be able to comfortably run five minutes at a time. If this schedule seems too challenging for you, start with the 30-Day Beginner Running Program in Part One of this book. If you find that this training schedule is advancing too quickly (and you're not signed up for a 5K just yet), you can stay on a week and repeat the workouts before moving on to the next week.

You don't have to do your runs on specific days; however, you should try not to run two days in a row. Either take a complete rest day or do cross-training (CT) on the days in between runs. Cross-training can be cycling, yoga, swimming, or any other activity (other than running) that you enjoy. Strength-training two to three times a week is also very beneficial for runners.

You should start each run with a 5 to 10-minute warm-up walk or jog. Finish up with a 5 to 10-minute cool-down walk or jog. Your run intervals should be done at an easy, conversational pace.

Look back to Chapter 12 for even more training and racing tips!

**Week 1:**
Day 1: Run 5 minutes, walk 1 min – repeat 3 times
Day 2: Rest or 30 min CT
Day 3: Run 6 minutes, walk 1 min – repeat 3 times
Day 4: Rest
Day 5: Run 7 minutes, walk 1 min – repeat 3 times
Day 6: Rest or 30 min CT
Day 7: Rest

**Week 2:**
Day 1: Run 7 minutes, walk 1 min – repeat 3 times
Day 2: Rest or 30 min CT
Day 3: Run 8 minutes, walk 1 min – repeat 3 times
Day 4: Rest
Day 5: Run 9 minutes mile, walk 1 min – repeat 3 times
Day 6: Rest or 30 min CT
Day 7: Rest

**Week 3:**
Day 1: Run 10 minutes, walk 1 min – repeat 2 times
Day 2: 30 min CT
Day 3: Run 12 minutes, walk 1 min – repeat 2 times
Day 4: Rest
Day 5: Run 13 minutes, walk 1 min – repeat 2 times
Day 6: Rest or 30 min CT
Day 7: Rest

**Week 4:**
Day 1: Run 15 minutes, walk 1 min - repeat 2 times
Day 2: 30 min CT
Day 3: Run 17 minutes, walk 1 min, run 7 min
Day 4: Rest
Day 5: Run 19 minutes, walk 1 min, run 7 min
Day 6: Rest or 30 min CT
Day 7: Rest

**Week 5:**
Day 1: Run 20 minutes, walk 1 min, run 6 min
Day 2: 30 min CT
Day 3: Run 24 minutes
Day 4: Rest
Day 5: Run 26 minutes
Day 6: Rest or 30 min CT
Day 7: Rest

**Week 6:**
Day 1: Run 28 minutes
Day 2: Rest or 30 min CT
Day 3: Run 30 minutes
Day 4: Rest
Day 5: Run 20 minutes
Day 6: Rest
Day 7: Race! Run 3.1 miles

## 10K Beginner Training Schedule

This six-week 10K training program is designed for beginner run/walkers who want to build up to running a 10K (6.2 miles). Ideally, to start this training program, you should be active a couple days a week and can run up to two miles. If you're not quite there, start with the 5K schedule.

**Long Runs (LR):** You're not training for a long distance event, but long runs will help you develop your stamina, which is important in 10K racing. You should do these runs at a comfortable, conversational pace. You should be able to breathe easily and talk in complete sentences. Your easy runs (ER) should also be done at this effort.

**Rest Days:** On rest days, you can take the day off or do some easy cross-training (CT), such as biking, swimming, yoga, strength training or another activity you enjoy.

**Week 1:**
Day 1: 30 min CT or Rest
Day 2: 2 miles ER
Day 3: 30 min CT or Rest
Day 4: 2 miles ER
Day 5: Rest
Day 6: 2 miles LR
Day 7: 2 miles brisk walk or Rest

**Week 2:**
Day 1: 30 min CT or Rest
Day 2: 2.5 miles ER
Day 3: 30 min CT or Rest
Day 4: 2.5 miles ER
Day 5: Rest
Day 6: 3 miles LR
Day 7: 2 miles brisk walk or Rest

**Week 3:**
Day 1: 30 min CT or Rest
Day 2: 3 miles ER
Day 3: 30 min CT or Rest
Day 4: 3 miles ER
Day 5: Rest
Day 6: 4 miles LR
Day 7: 2 miles brisk walk or Rest

**Week 4:**
Day 1: 30 min CT or Rest
Day 2: 3 miles ER
Day 3: 30 min CT or Rest
Day 4: 4 miles ER
Day 5: Rest
Day 6: 5 miles LR
Day 7: 2 miles brisk walk or Rest

**Week 5:**
Day 1: 30 min CT or Rest
Day 2: 3 miles ER
Day 3: 30 min CT or Rest
Day 4: 4 miles ER
Day 5: Rest
Day 6: 4 miles LR
Day 7: 2 miles brisk walk or Rest

**Week 6:**
Day 1: 3 miles ER
Day 2: 30 min CT or Rest
Day 3: 3 miles ER
Day 4: Rest
Day 5: 2 miles ER
Day 6: Rest
Day 7: Race day!

## Half-Marathon Beginner Schedule

This 12-week half marathon training program is designed to help you run/walk to the finish line of a half marathon (13.1 miles). To start this plan, you should have been run/walking for at least two months and should have a base mileage of about 8 to 10 miles per week. If you're not quite ready for that, start with the 10K beginner schedule.

This beginner training schedule is a run/walk program, so your workout instructions will be displayed in run/walk intervals. The first number displayed is the amount of minutes to run and the second number is the amount to walk. So, for example, 3/1 means run for 3 minutes, then walk for 1 minute.

If you can already run 2 to 3 miles continuously, you can ignore the run/walk or walk instructions and run for the indicated distances.

You should start each run with a 5 to 10-minute warm-up walk or jog. Finish up with a 5 to 10-minute cool-down walk or jog. Your run intervals should be done at an easy, conversational pace.

**Scheduling:** You don't have to do your runs on specific days; however, make sure you don't run every day. You want to mix in some rest days and cross-training (CT). Cross-training can be walking, biking, swimming, strength training or any other activity (other than running) that you enjoy. You'll most likely want to do your long runs on Saturday or Sunday, when you'll have more time.

**Week 1:**
Day 1: 2 miles - 2/1 run/walk intervals
Day 2: 30 min CT or Rest
Day 3: 2.5 miles - 2/1 run/walk intervals
Day 4: 30 min CT or Rest
Day 5: Rest
Day 6: 3 miles (long run) - 2/1 run/walk intervals
Day 7: 2 miles (recovery walk)

**Week 2:**
Day 1: 2 miles - 2/1 run/walk intervals
Day 2: 30 min CT or rest
Day 3: 3 miles - 2/1 run/walk intervals
Day 4: 30 min CT or rest
Day 5: Rest
Day 6: 4 miles (long run) - 2/1 run/walk intervals
Day 7: 2.5 miles (recovery walk)

**Week 3:**
Day 1: 2.5 miles - 2/1 run/walk intervals
Day 2: 30 min CT or rest
Day 3: 3 miles - 2/1 run/walk intervals
Day 4: 30 min CT or rest
Day 5: Rest
Day 6: 5 miles (long run) - 2/1 run/walk intervals
Day 7: 2 miles (recovery walk)

**Week 4:**
Day 1: 2.5 miles - 3/1 run/walk intervals
Day 2: 30 min CT or rest
Day 3: 3 miles - 3/1 run/walk intervals
Day 4: 30 min CT or rest
Day 5: Rest
Day 6: 6 miles (long run) - 3/1 run/walk intervals
Day 7: 2 miles (recovery walk)

**Week 5:**
Day 1: 3 miles - 3/1 run/walk intervals
Day 2: 30 min CT or rest
Day 3: 3 miles - 3/1 run/walk intervals
Day 4: 30 min CT or rest
Day 5: Rest
Day 6: 7 miles (long run) - 3/1 run/walk intervals
Day 7: 3 miles (recovery walk)

**Week 6:**
Day 1: 3 miles - 3/1 run/walk intervals
Day 2: 30 min CT or rest
Day 3: 4 miles - 3/1 run/walk intervals
Day 4: 30 min CT or rest
Day 5: Rest
Day 6: 8 miles (long run) - 3/1 run/walk intervals
Day 7: 3 miles (recovery walk)

**Week 7:**
Day 1: 3 miles - 3/1 run/walk intervals
Day 2: 30 min CT or rest
Day 3: 4 miles - 3/1 run/walk intervals
Day 4: 30 min CT or rest
Day 5: Rest
Day 6: 9 miles (long run) - 3/1 run/walk intervals
Day 7: 3 miles easy (recovery walk)

**Week 8:**
Day 1: 4 miles - 3/1 run/walk intervals
Day 2: 30 min CT or rest
Day 3: 3 miles- 3/1 run/walk intervals
Day 4: 30 min CT or rest
Day 5: Rest
Day 6: 10 miles (long run) - 3/1 run/walk intervals
Day 7: 3 miles EZ (recovery walk)

**Week 9:**
Day 1: 4 miles - 3/1 run/walk intervals
Day 2: 30 min CT or rest
Day 3: 4 miles - 3/1 run/walk intervals
Day 4: 30 min CT or rest
Day 5: Rest
Day 6: 11 miles (long run) - 3/1 run/walk intervals
Day 7: 3 mi EZ (recovery walk)

**Week 10:**
Day 1: 4 miles - 3/1 run/walk intervals
Day 2: 30 min CT or rest
Day 3: 3 miles - 3/1 run/walk intervals
Day 4: 30 min CT or rest
Day 5: Rest
Day 6: 12 mi (long run) - 3/1 run/walk intervals
Day 7: 3 mi EZ (recovery walk)

**Week 11:**
Day 1: 30 min CT or rest
Day 2: 3 miles- 3/1 run/walk intervals
Day 3: 30 min CT or rest
Day 4:  3 miles- 3/1 run/walk intervals
Day 5: Rest
Day 6: 5 miles (long run) - 3/1 run/walk intervals
Day 7: 2.5 miles (recovery walk)

**Week 12:**
Day 1: 2 miles - 3/1 run/walk intervals
Day 2: 30 min CT or rest
Day 3: Rest
Day 4: 20 minutes - 3/1 run/walk intervals
Day 5: Rest
Day 6: (day before race): Walk 20 minutes
Day 7: RACE!

## **Marathon Training Beginner Schedule**

This 20-week marathon training program is designed to help you run/walk to the finish line of your marathon (26.2 miles). To start this plan, you should have been run/walking for at least six months and should have a base mileage of about 12 to 15 miles per week.

This beginner training schedule is a run/walk program, so your workout instructions will be displayed in run/walk intervals. The first number displayed is the amount of minutes to run and the second number is the amount to walk. So, for example, 3/1 means run for 3 minutes, then walk for 1 minute. If 3/1 intervals start to get too easy during your training, you can shoot for 4/1 or 5/1 intervals.

If you can already run 3 miles continuously, you can ignore the run/walk or walk instructions and run for the indicated distances.

You should start each run with a 5 to 10-minute warm-up walk or jog. Finish up with a 5 to 10-minute cool-down walk or jog. Your run intervals should be done at an easy, conversational pace. You should finish your runs with overall stretching.

You don't have to do your runs on specific days; however, make sure you don't run every day. You want to mix in some rest days and cross-training (CT). Cross-training can be walking, yoga, Pilates, cycling, rowing, swimming, or any activity (other than running) that you enjoy. You'll most likely want to do your long runs on Saturday or Sunday, when you'll have more time.

**Week 1:**
Day 1: 2 miles - 2/1 run/walk intervals
Day 2: 30 minutes CT
Day 3: 3 miles - 2/1 run/walk intervals
Day 4: 30 minutes CT or Rest
Day 5: Rest
Day 6: 4 miles (long run) - 2/1 run/walk intervals
Day 7: 2 miles (recovery walk)

**Week 2:**
Day 1: 3 miles - 2/1 run/walk intervals
Day 2: 30 minutes CT
Day 3: 3 miles - 2/1 run/walk intervals
Day 4: 30 minutes CT or Rest
Day 5: Rest
Day 6: 4 miles (long run) - 2/1 run/walk intervals
Day 7: 2.5 miles (recovery walk)

**Week 3:**
Day 1: 3 miles - 2/1 run/walk intervals
Day 2: 30 minutes CT
Day 3: 3 miles - 2/1 run/walk intervals
Day 4: 30 minutes CT or Rest
Day 5: Rest
Day 6: 5 miles (long run) - 2/1 run/walk intervals
Day 7: 2 miles (recovery walk)

**Week 4:**
Day 1: 3 miles - 3/1 run/walk intervals
Day 2: 30 minutes CT
Day 3: 3 miles - 3/1 run/walk intervals
Day 4: 30 minutes CT or Rest
Day 5: Rest
Day 6: 6 miles (long run) - 3/1 run/walk intervals
Day 7: 2 miles (recovery walk)

**Week 5:**
Day 1: 3 miles - 3/1 run/walk intervals
Day 2: 30 minutes CT
Day 3: 3 miles - 3/1 run/walk intervals
Day 4: 30 minutes CT or Rest
Day 5: Rest
Day 6: 7 miles (long run) - 3/1 run/walk intervals
Day 7: 3 miles (recovery walk)

**Week 6:**
Day 1: 3 miles - 3/1 run/walk intervals
Day 2: 30 minutes CT
Day 3: 4 miles - 3/1 run/walk intervals
Day 4: 30 minutes CT or Rest
Day 5: Rest
Day 6: 8 miles (long run) - 3/1 run/walk intervals
Day 7: 3 miles (recovery walk)

**Week 7:**
Day 1: 3 miles - 3/1 run/walk intervals
Day 2: 40 minutes CT
Day 3: 4 miles - 3/1 run/walk intervals

Day 4: 30 minutes CT or Rest
Day 5: Rest
Day 6: 9 miles (long run) - 3/1 run/walk intervals
Day 7: 3 miles EZ (recovery walk)

**Week 8:**
Day 1: 4 miles - 3/1 run/walk intervals
Day 2: 40 minutes CT
Day 3: 3 miles- 3/1 run/walk intervals
Day 4: 30 minutes CT or Rest
Day 5: Rest
Day 6: 10 miles (long run) - 3/1 run/walk intervals
Day 7: 3 miles EZ (recovery walk)

**Week 9:**
Day 1: 3 miles - 3/1 run/walk intervals
Day 2: 40 minutes CT
Day 3: 4 miles - 3/1 run/walk intervals
Day 4: 30 minutes CT or Rest
Day 5: Rest
Day 6: 12 miles (long run) - 3/1 run/walk intervals
Day 7: 3 mi EZ (recovery walk)

**Week 10:**
Day 1: 4 miles - 3/1 run/walk intervals
Day 2: 45 minutes CT
Day 3: 4 miles - 3/1 run/walk intervals
Day 4: 30 minutes CT or Rest
Day 5: Rest
Day 6: 8 mi (long run) - 3/1 run/walk intervals
Day 7: 3 mi EZ (recovery walk)

**Week 11:**
Day 1: 3 miles- 3/1 run/walk intervals
Day 2: 45 minutes CT
Day 3: 3 miles- 3/1 run/walk intervals
Day 4: 30 minutes CT or Rest
Day 5: Rest
Day 6: 14 miles (long run) - 3/1 run/walk intervals
Day 7: 2.5 miles (recovery walk)

**Week 12:**
Day 1: 4 miles - 3/1 run/walk intervals
Day 2: 45 minutes CT
Day 3: 3 miles- 3/1 run/walk intervals
Day 4: 30 minutes CT or Rest
Day 5: Rest
Day 6: 10 miles (long run) - 3/1 run/walk intervals
Day 7: 3 miles (recovery walk)

**Week 13:**
Day 1: 4 miles - 3/1 run/walk intervals
Day 2: 45 minutes CT
Day 3: 3 miles- 3/1 run/walk intervals
Day 4: 30 minutes CT or Rest
Day 5: Rest
Day 6: 15 miles (long run) - 3/1 run/walk intervals
Day 7: 3 miles (recovery walk)

**Week 14:**
Day 1: 4 miles - 3/1 run/walk intervals
Day 2: 45 minutes CT
Day 3: 3 miles- 3/1 run/walk intervals

Day 4: 30 minutes CT or Rest
Day 5: Rest
Day 6: 10 miles (long run) - 3/1 run/walk intervals
Day 7: 3 miles (recovery walk)

**Week 15:**
Day 1: 4 miles - 3/1 run/walk intervals
Day 2: 45 minutes CT
Day 3: 4 miles- 3/1 run/walk intervals
Day 4: 30 minutes CT or Rest
Day 5: Rest
Day 6: 16 miles (long run) - 3/1 run/walk intervals
Day 7: 3 miles (recovery walk)

**Week 16:**
Day 1: 4 miles - 3/1 run/walk intervals
Day 2: 45 minutes CT
Day 3: 3 miles- 3/1 run/walk intervals
Day 4: 30 minutes CT or Rest
Day 5: Rest
Day 6: 12 miles (long run) - 3/1 run/walk intervals
Day 7: 2.5 miles (recovery walk)

**Week 17:**
Day 1: 4 miles - 3/1 run/walk intervals
Day 2: 45 minutes CT
Day 3: 3 miles- 3/1 run/walk intervals
Day 4: 30 minutes CT or Rest
Day 5: Rest
Day 6: 18 to 20 miles (long run) - 3/1 run/walk intervals
Day 7: 2.5 miles (recovery walk)

**Week 18:**

Day 1: 4 miles - 3/1 run/walk intervals
Day 2: 45 minutes CT
Day 3: 3 miles- 3/1 run/walk intervals
Day 4: 30 minutes CT or Rest
Day 5: Rest
Day 6: 12 miles (long run) - 3/1 run/walk intervals
Day 7: 2.5 miles (recovery walk)

**Week 19:**

Day 1: 45 minutes CT
Day 2: 3 miles- 3/1 run/walk intervals
Day 3: 30 minutes CT or Rest
Day 4: 2 miles- 3/1 run/walk intervals
Day 5: Rest
Day 6: 6 miles (long run) - 3/1 run/walk intervals
Day 7: 2.5 miles (recovery walk)

**Week 20:**

Day 1: 3 miles - 3/1 run/walk intervals
Day 2: 30 minutes - 3/1 run/walk intervals
Day 3: Rest
Day 4: 20 minutes - 3/1 run/walk intervals
Day 5: Rest
Day 6 (day before race): Walk 20 minutes
Day 7: RACE!

For even more training schedules for all distances and levels, go to run-for-good.com/category/running/training-schedules/

## Suggested Reading/Bibliography

I've referred to all of these books in *Run for Good* and highly recommend them to anyone trying to establish a running habit, or make any healthy, positive changes. Like this book, you can read (or listen to) them for advice on getting started with and maintaining a new habit and for motivation and inspiration on how to live a more positive and fulfilling life.

Carter, Christine, Ph.D. *The Sweet Spot: How to Find Your Groove at Home and Work*. New York: Ballantine Books, 2015

Doepker, Derek. *The Healthy Habit Revolution: Create Better Habits in Five Minutes a Day*, Createspace, 2014

Duhigg, Charles. *The Power of Habit: Why We Do What We Do in Life and Business*. New York: Random House, 2012

Guise, Stephen. *Mini Habits: Smaller Habits, Bigger Results*. Createspace, 2013

Huffington, Arianna. *Thrive: The Third Metric to Redefining Success and Creating a Life of Well-Being, Wisdom, and Wonder*. New York: Random House, 2014

Loehr, Jim and Tony Schwartz. *The Power of Full Engagement: Managing Energy, Not Time, Is the Key to High Performance and Personal Renewal*. New York: Free Press, 2003

Rubin, Gretchen. *Better Than Before: Mastering the Habits of our Everyday Lives*. New York: Random House, 2015

Vanderkam, Laura. *I Know How She Does It: How Successful Women Make the Most of Their Time*. New York: Portfolio/Penguin, 2016

## About the Author

Christine Many Luff lives and breathes running. Her passion for the sport filters through many aspects of her life—as a fitness writer, avid runner, certified running coach and personal trainer.

As a coach for the Leukemia and Lymphoma Society's Team in Training (TNT) running team in New York City since 2003, Christine has trained thousands of runners to cross the finish lines of dozens of full and half-marathons. She has run 13 marathons and countless other races. A big advocate of youth running, Christine also coaches her kids' track & field team. Some of her favorite running moments have been watching kids cross the finish line of their first race.

As a health and fitness writer/editor, Christine has held staff positions at various magazines and websites and has written for numerous sports and fitness publications and websites. She resides in New Jersey with her husband and two kids.

CPSIA information can be obtained
at www.ICGtesting.com
Printed in the USA
FSHW021104281118
54089FS